Adore Your Lifestyle

A healthy eating & lifestyle guide for every **body**

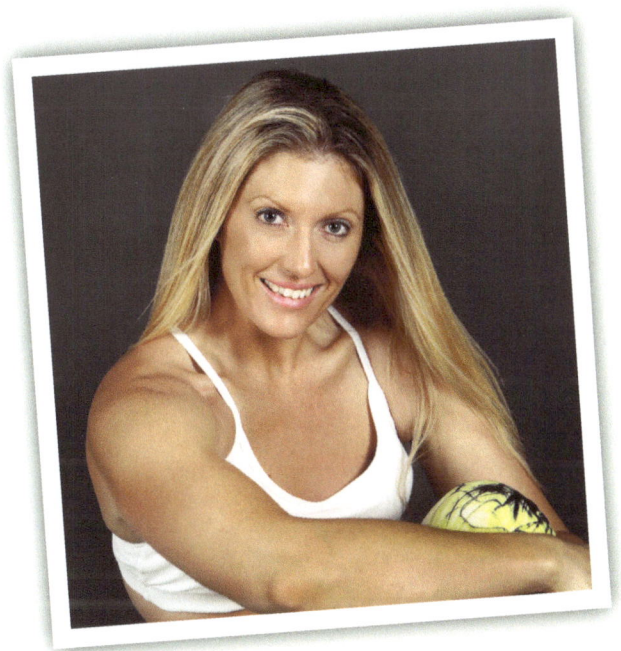

Cat Adora

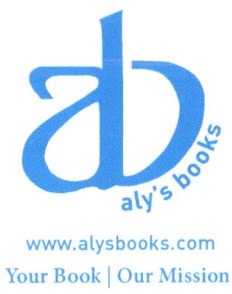

www.alysbooks.com
Your Book | Our Mission

Adore Your Lifestyle
— A healthy eating & lifestyle guide for every body

Copyright © Cat Adora

First Edition 2015
Published by Aly's Books

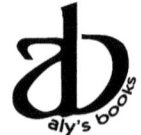

www.alysbooks.com
Your Book | Our Mission

Edited by Irrefutable Proof
www.irrefutable-proof.com

Edited by writelinda
Twitter: @writelinda

Designed by Fish Biscuit
fishbiscuitdesign.com.au

All rights reserved. No part of this book may be reproduced or transmitted in any form or by any means, electronic, mechanical, photocopying or otherwise without the prior permission of the publisher.

ISBN: 978 0 9944015 1 9

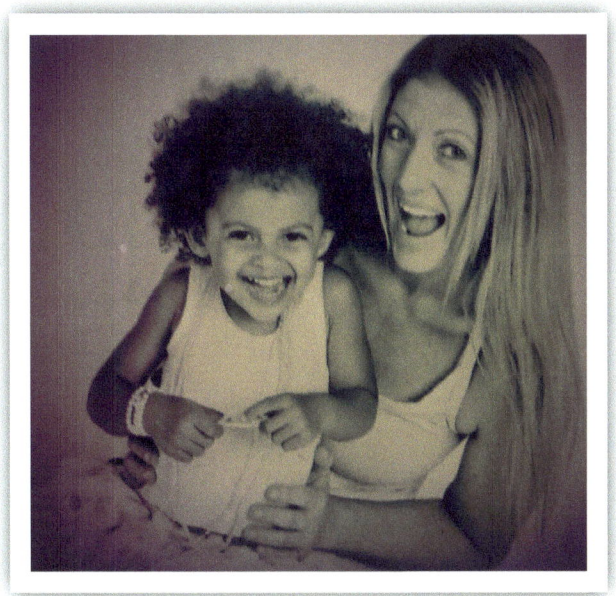

This book is for my amazing and absolutely incredible daughter who inspires me every single day and continually shows me the importance of looking beyond what the eyes can see – looking at life with the innocence and appreciation of a child and simply loving and *living* life.

For the health of her generation and the generations to come. For my Zen who believes in me beyond measure, and for my Grandfather – without his continued love, support and devotion this chapter in my life would not have been possible.

Cat Adora

Contents

Where it all began... 6
Helpful Tools for the Kitchen 10
Why use pink Himalayan salt 10
Why cook with raw, cold pressed coconut oil 10
Steer away from starchy foods where possible 10
Why I love to use a non-stick sandwich press for most of my cooking 10

Adore Nature's Milks
Almond Milk 11
Coconut Milk – the milk of life 11
Make your own LSA 12
Natural Alternative Protein Powders 12

Adore Juices and Smoothies
Cold Press Juices and Smoothies 13
Directions for all juice recipies 13
Smoothies 14
The Green Machine 14
Antioxidant Booster 14
Berry Bliss 14
Nature's Pina Colada 15
Fresh Breathe Juice 15
Midday Power Kick 15
The Carrot Kiss - eyesight and brain function improver 15
The Calmer 15
Pineapple, Lemon, Ginger Juice 16
Red Divine 16
Skin Glow and Repair Juice 16
Immune Defence Shot 17
Daily Energizer 17
Avocado Smoothie 17

Adore Mornings
Eggs and Omelettes 18
Folded Egg with Fresh Basil, Chilli and Cherry tomato stir-fry, Coconut fried mushrooms and cooling avocado 18
Warm Egg Salad 19
Kale and Feta Omelette 19
Easy Omelette - sandwich press style 19
Egg and Vege Fry Up 20
Bok Choy, Fresh Chilli, Herb and Kumara Eggs 20

Morning meal time
Avocado Muesli 21
Raw Choc Granola 22
Morning POW 22
Morning Rainbow Oats 22
Blueberry Pancakes 23
Layered Tropical fruits with pistachio nibs 23
Easy Savoury Pancakes 24
Paw Paw and Fresh Mint Fruit Salad 24
Banana, Nut Milk and Morning Seed Medley 24
Smashed Avocado and Jacket Kumara 25
Banana Strawberry Smoothie Bowl 25

Adore Main Meals
Raw plant-based whole foods 26
Raw Shaved Savoy and Zucchini noodles with Fresh Garlic Herb Sauce, Crispy Yam and Okra 27
Avocado Rice Salad 27
Crispy Tofu and Chilli Stir Fry 28
African Mediterranean Inspired Veggies 28
Warm Sweet Potato and Zucchini Medley 29
Indian-Inspired Spice-Infused Lentils (or lean beef) and Fresh Herb Cabbage Cradles 29
Black Rice, Broccoli, Black Bean (or beef) and Sweet Potato Medley 30
Zucchini Fritters 30
Spicy Anaheim Pepper Bruschetta – also known as chiayo chilli or banana chilli 31
Thai-Inspired Shredded Organic Chicken or Tofu Soup 31
Crunchy Coconut Prawn heads with folded egg, organic cottage or goat cheese and pan fried cherry tomato 32
Raw Pad Thai with Creamy Cashew Dressing 33
Warm Rainbow Carrot Medley 33
Plantain Skewers with Okra, Poached Crisped Yam, Red Peppers, Raw Honey and Himalayan salt 34
Pizza of Health 35
Spicy Tuna Bolognese 35
Coconut Pumpkin Soup 36

Adore Salads
Avocado and Beetroot Salad with Eggplant Crisps 37
Deconstructed Bruschetta Yellow Bell Pepper Boats 38
Golden Beet, Fresh Basil and Cashew Salad 38
Warm Kumara and Golden Beet Salad 39
Purple Cabbage Salad Bowls and Wraps 39
Green Sprout and Lime Salad 40
Healing Herb and Mixed Kale Salad 40
Spiralized Carrot Grilled Chicken and Sesame Salad 41
Zucchini Tahini Salad 41
Egyptian Inspired Barley, Fennel and Cucumber Salad 42
Easy Summer Cooler Salad 42
Warm Chickpea Rainbow Salad 43
Tabouleh Avocado Boats 43
Avocado and Sweet Basil Salad 43
Pomegranate, Purple Cabbage and Fresh crispy Kale Salad 44
Balsamic, Feta and Cos Lettuce Salad 44
Vietnam on a plate 45
Watercress, Cucumber and Spring Water Tuna Salad 45
Kale Garden Salad and Avocado 46
Curly Carrot, Sunflower Sprout and Roasted Peanut Salad 46

Adore Dips, Dressings and Sauces

Guacamole	47
Creamy Cashew Dressing	47
African Inspired Hot Chilli Dipping Sauce	48
Tahini	48
Garlic Dipping Sauce	48
Lemon Citrus Vinaigrette	49
Easy Herb and Mustard Seed Dressing with Lime	49
Pesto	49
Smashed Avocado	49
Mango and Pomegranate Dressing	50
Sweet and Spicy Chilli Sauce	50
Coriander Lime Chilli Dressing	50
Fresh Tomato and Bay leaf Sauce	51

Adore Snacks and Starters

Fruit Sticks	52
Power and Energy Balls	52
Carrot, Ginger and Walnut Energy Balls	52
Green Power Energy Balls	53
Apple Peanut Stacks	53
Pineapple Paradise Slushie	53
Raw Dark Choc Fruit and Nut Protein Balls	54
Pear, Walnut and Mint Refresher	54
Sweet Potato Wedges, Yam and Kumara Fries with Garlic Dipping Sauce	55
Banana, Cacao nib and Peanut Bites	55
Red Grapefruit, Raw Macadamia and Mint Revitaliser	56
Rosemary Mint Hummus	56
Rainbow Veggie Sticks	57
Soft Raw Caramel Chews	57
Tahini and Tomato Bites	57
Pineapple, Chilli and Mint Ice Pops	58
Creamy Coconut, Tangerine and Turmeric Ice Lickers	58
Raw Rocky Road	58
Mango and Rasperry Ice Blocks	59
Watermelon and Lychee Lickers or Passionfruit and Watermelon Ice Pops	59
Raw 'Cobana' Bombs	59
Zucchini Rolls with Creamy Pine Nut Cheese	60
Raw Choc Protein Balls	60

Snacks To Have On Hand

Instant and Amazing Snack – to kick those sugar cravings	61
Toasted Garlic and Eggplant Crisps	61
Nut Crunch Slice	61

Adore Dessert

Red Ruby Sorbet	62
Strawberry Banana Delight Cream Bombs	62
Raw Blueberry 'Ice-Cream' Cheesecake	63
Plum Sorbet	63
Raw Choc Crunch Mousse	64
Raw Carrot Cake	64
Cookie Dough	65
Salty-Sweet Raw Banana Delight Cream	65
Licorice Delight Cream	65
Raw Strawberry Cheesecake	66
Red Dragon Fruit Delight Cream	66
Dragon Fruit drink cubes	67
Raw Mint Choc Slice	67
Fig Delight Cream	67
Warm Plantain Fingers - my little taste of Fiji	68
Raw Cherry Ripe Slice	68
Deconstructed Raw Banoffee Pie	69
Carambola Star Fruit or Fuji Persimmon and Fresh Fig Chocolate Fondue	69
Honey Comb Rhubarb Crumble Loaf	70
Frosty Fruit Royale	71
Papaya Bliss balls	71
Summer Paw Paw Pleasure Boats	72
Chocolate Coated Banana and Cinnamon Pops	72
Raw Coconut Rough Ice cream with Broken Chocolate	73

Adore Teas, Herbs and Useful Uses

Herbs and spices to have on hand	74
Oils and natural dressings to have on hand	74
Natural Cough Remedy Tea	74
Vietnamese Inspired Sore Throat Cure Tea	74
Healthy Heart Tea	75
Orange Comfort Tea	75
Peppermint Tea Naturally – The Stomach Settler	75
Turmeric Tea	76
Essential Warm Lemon Water	76

My Love for Herbs and Spices 77

Adore Life 78

Adore Health... a healthy life starts with healthy thoughts 79

Adore Fitness

Some excellent Body Weight Exercises that I live by	80
What my typical day looks like – a guide to daily healthy eating and lifestyle	82

Endorsements 85

Special Mention 88

Dedications 89

Glossary 90

Disclaimer	92

Where it all began...

Many of us are thrown challenges that seem impossible to face, let alone walk through.

In July of 2011, I gave birth to the most beautiful baby girl I could ever have imagined – my angel, my joy, my sunshine!

I went through a very difficult time throughout my pregnancy and gained a whopping 42kg - taking me to a total of 115kg. I could have easily found myself staring down a dark and gloomy path to my future, one of being grossly overweight, accepting that this was now me, but that is NOT who I am.

I will always see the best in life in any circumstance, be it good or bad. I don't like to take the easy way out, and accepting 'what is' was not an option for me. Coming from a background in dance, I had always been athletic, energetic, healthy and active. So I began my journey back to fitness the moment I was out of hospital.

I made my mind up then and there, that there was no turning back. There was no quitting. I would see this journey through to the end no matter how long it took. Once my mind was made up, my body followed.

I began slowly at first, with low-impact exercise. Gradually, as my body healed and my strength returned, I began to make progress. Amazingly, less than eight weeks after birth, I had lost 18kg, all thanks to healthy eating and the low impact exercise I was doing – walking and swimming! In late September 2011, ten weeks after giving birth, I began taking one-hour hypoxi training sessions, and I walked an hour each way to my sessions, pushing my baby in the pram.
By early February 2012, just over four months later, I had lost another 24kg, totalling a massive 42kg weight loss. I'd done it! And more importantly, it had only taken me a little less than 20 weeks! My determination, total commitment and consistency were paying off.

I endured a whirlwind of experiences in the remainder of 2012. A huge move interstate, moving between suburbs once there and later joining a mothers' fitness group that ended in a nightmare experience – it all added up to a very trying time. I was unsettled and frustrated, and along with dealing with several stressful personal situations in my life, I found I had a slight weight gain.

I've been through it all, but I NEVER gave up. I have had that draining feeling of being 'stuck-in-a-rut', feeling like I was going around in circles, busting out my all to try and find the kind of training I was hungry for, giving a hundred per cent the whole time but feeling like nothing worked.

Even with all this, I gained deep insight into my own knowledge and understanding of nutrition, health and fitness.

I found I was constantly seeking the next challenge, I wanted more. I had seen the results my body had achieved and I wanted to go further, be stronger, fitter!

I encountered negative input along the way. I was being told that I would never be able to lose all the weight I had gained. Several people told me I would never get back to the way I was, and I was even told to consider a tummy tuck by a fitness instructor! I defied the odds and never allowed anyone to sway me from my goal. It only made me more determined.

February 2013 started me on a fresh fitness path with body sculpting sessions – I was hooked from the word go!

Again I saw rapid results within just eight weeks. I know this was also due to my dedication, commitment and consistency, along with a stronger understanding of nutrition. I began to create and follow my own nutrition and eating plan, and in April 2013 I decided to join a gym. This was something I had long avoided, as gyms can often be intimidating.

I started taking body pump classes and boxing. I lost another 4kg. My eating and exercise strategies were having a positive effect on my lifestyle, and it drove me to research and learn more. In May 2013, for the first time in my life, I began to lift weights. I quickly discovered that this was the missing link in my health and fitness journey.

Four months later, in September 2013, and at an overall total weight loss of 52kg, reaching

18 percent body fat, (yes, now in the athlete bracket – 20 percent or less body fat, woohoo!) this was the new me!

I wasn't always fit and strong – both physically and mentally. Some days I found myself in tears because it was all too much. I was raising my daughter under very difficult circumstances, with very little support, and in a place where I hated how I looked and how I felt. I have battled and fought the mental fears and the physical doubts and obstacles. I have struggled with the embarrassment and inner torment that being overweight can bring. I have felt the claws of depression close in on me. I have fallen down many times, almost to the point where bitter defeat felt better than sweet victory. I have stared down the barrel of humiliation. I have felt the agony and exhaustion that getting up to try and carry on, over and over again, can bring. I have stood at the door of hopelessness...

The journey has not been easy but I survived. I never gave up. I defied my impossible. I now know what it means to be strong mentally, not just physically. My story is still being written. Struggles and obstacles don't go away – you learn to tackle them differently and you learn how to fight your personal battles. My choice to fight back has greatly influenced my daughter, and for that reason alone, I am so grateful for the struggle that taught me how to rise above all.

What do I do, to stay motivated? How do I get up daily and push on when I feel like I can't? What do I do to beat the rut and the many excuses? I stay THANKFUL! How often we forget just how much we have and how lucky we are! I am blessed with two arms and two legs, I am healthy, and I have no excuses, so why wouldn't I get up and give each day, a day that I can never get back again, my best and my all? I look at circumstance – it is only temporary! YOU have the choice to let it consume you, or to use what is happening in your life to your benefit, to overcome.

Look at situations with the attitude of 'I'm going to get through this the best way I can' and take it step by step, instead of asking 'why me?' The battle of the mind is fierce. It is a daily discipline. But

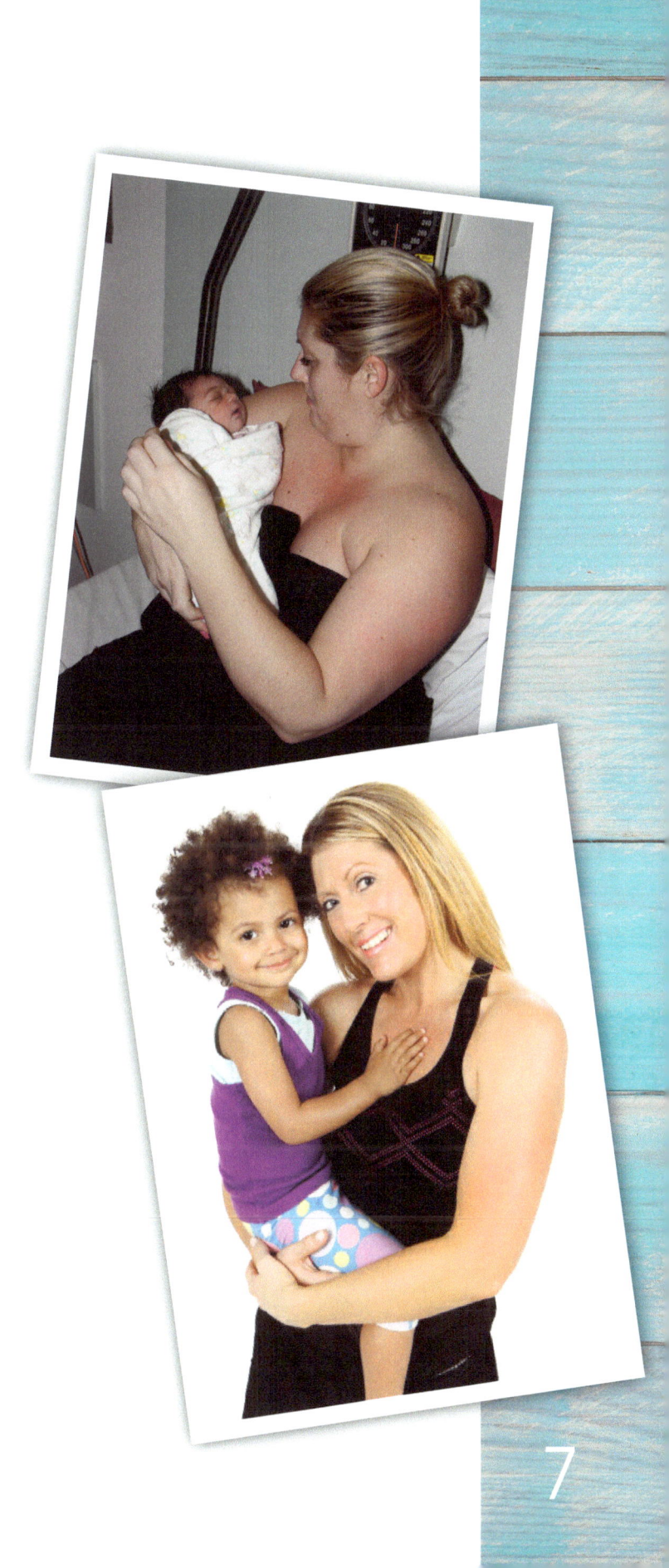

it is also a privilege, for that is where we mould and form our strength. It is not easy – the struggle is very real. But ask yourself, why am I making excuses? Why am I complaining? Why have I set my frame of mind to think it's too hard, or to believe I just don't have the time?

We are all in that same boat, but I tell you if you want something enough you will find a way to get it, no matter what! Don't look at the road and say 'I can't', look at the journey and say "I'm willing and I'm wanting." Then take the first step… and JUST START.

Start with small changes – exercise for 30 minutes, 45 minutes, an hour and so on. Don't compare yourself to anyone. Make a decision to choose health and happiness; it is a choice. Did you know the ability to make choices is a GIFT not a right? I keep my home full of healthy food, avoiding temptation. I am at a point now where I only want to eat food that will heal me, not food that will harm me. It is a process, but you begin to realise it is not at all about diet. It's about LIFEstyle and optimum health. I don't ever think that I'm missing out, I am thankful that I CAN eat for my health, that the choice is so freely available to us. My daughter is a huge motivator for me to keep fit. Our children watch what we do, and do what we do. Life is a gift and that's how I choose to live it, daily.

Nothing is handed to us on a platter. We have to get up and we have to fight for what we want. YOU have to do it because no one else can do it for you. This is what I realised...and this was my wake up call.

A lot of people want it, but they don't want to put the hard work in to get it. Then they complain when they don't look the way they want to, or don't get the results they are after.

I didn't want to be a statistic – the battles in my mind were tearing me apart, pulling me in all directions. I was angry, frustrated, embarrassed, overwhelmed, feeling defeated, but I also began to realise something. "Hey Cat, you have no excuse to be like this, no matter what is being thrown at you or what you have to face, your choices right here and now will decide your future."

I always thought about people starving in other countries too, and how much of a contradiction it is to be in such a physical state when people all over the world don't even have FOOD, let alone all the other daily essentials. I have a responsibility to myself, to my health, to my wellbeing and state of mind to look after my body, my health and my life! You can't rely on other people to get you over the line, you have to GET UP and start putting the effort in. If it were that easy, there wouldn't be any need for it in the first place.

I was thrown into the deep end from the word go. Tragic personal circumstances found me suddenly facing a harsh reality. A reality that first time mothers should never have to face. I didn't have any of the support around me that most first time mothers have. Those days were some of the hardest of my life.

I had no transport, so I had to walk for hours just to do a grocery shop, all while pushing my newborn baby in pram and carrying a massive load of shopping – it was crazy.

I look back and am still amazed at how far I have come. The immense amount of stress I was under, all the more intense while raising a new life. Sometimes it was almost too much to bear. Yet at our lowest points, if we choose to look, there is light shining through the gaps, just waiting for us to burst in head on at full speed, even when it feels absolutely impossible.

Don't look at the road and say 'I can't', look at the journey and say 'I'm willing and I'm wanting', and then take the first step and JUST START.

I found something I was excited about – I found an interest, a passion, and that is how I pulled myself out of the pit I was in. I had something to look forward to, to motivate me, to push me on, to be accountable for, to work towards, to beat and to fight for. It is one thing for someone to tell you to be mentally tough, but it's another thing entirely when you're suddenly thrust into situations you have no control over. It's draining.

It's a daily choice, and it's not easy but it does get easier. The hardest part is starting! You are upending your life from bad to better, and it will take time, so if you expect an overnight miracle you're setting yourself up for shattered expectations. It has to be a daily process. You can speed things up by jumping in the deep end, that's what I did. I figure if you're going to do something, why not do it all the way and with everything it takes from the word go? Plunge in, dive head first, there's no dipping in a hesitant toe to check how cold the water is, no way. I think that's the thing most people find the hardest. Really it comes back to HOW BAD DO YOU WANT IT? Small changes daily are great, and a positive start on the road to change for better health and wellbeing, but I'm the sort of person that when faced with a challenge, I charge at it with all I have. Don't get me wrong, I have fallen over many times, but I always get back up. Failure is just another lesson learned, never a loss, because failure means I am learning. I look at it as a way of finding the successful road that will take me to the heights I am aiming for. "Courage is not the failure to recognise fear; it is the refusal to accept its offer."

Above all, being disciplined is what is necessary for triumph. Get rid of the excuses – there will always be something to complain about, some reason not to do what you set out to do, but there is always a stronger positive, something to be thankful for that outweighs all negatives. I wasn't happy with being comfortable and not changing. I accepted the challenge because I was desperate for change and I'd had enough! For most of us, the battle starts in our heads.

My story is all about defying the impossible, going after your dreams no matter how hard it may seem and never giving up. I hope all who read about my journey will find great inspiration, and realise we ALL have the potential and ability to better

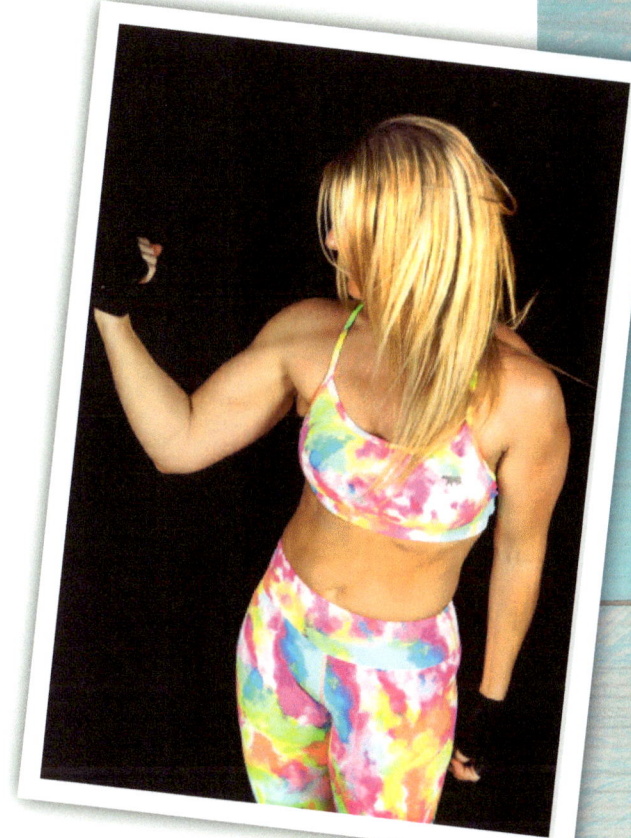

ourselves no matter the obstacle, no matter the impossibilities.

I am not there yet, my fitness journey is far from over. It is still being written.
It continues to take me to even greater heights than I ever could have imagined. I'm now fiercely training and competing in the sport of Olympic weight lifting, recently winning my first ever competition. The future is endless opportunity! As each goal is conquered I welcome new and greater challenges, but getting to where I am today is nothing short of a decision and a choice that I made.

My story doesn't have to be unique – it can be your story too. Your story, with your goals, your challenges and your successes.

Adore Your Lifestyle
Cat Adora

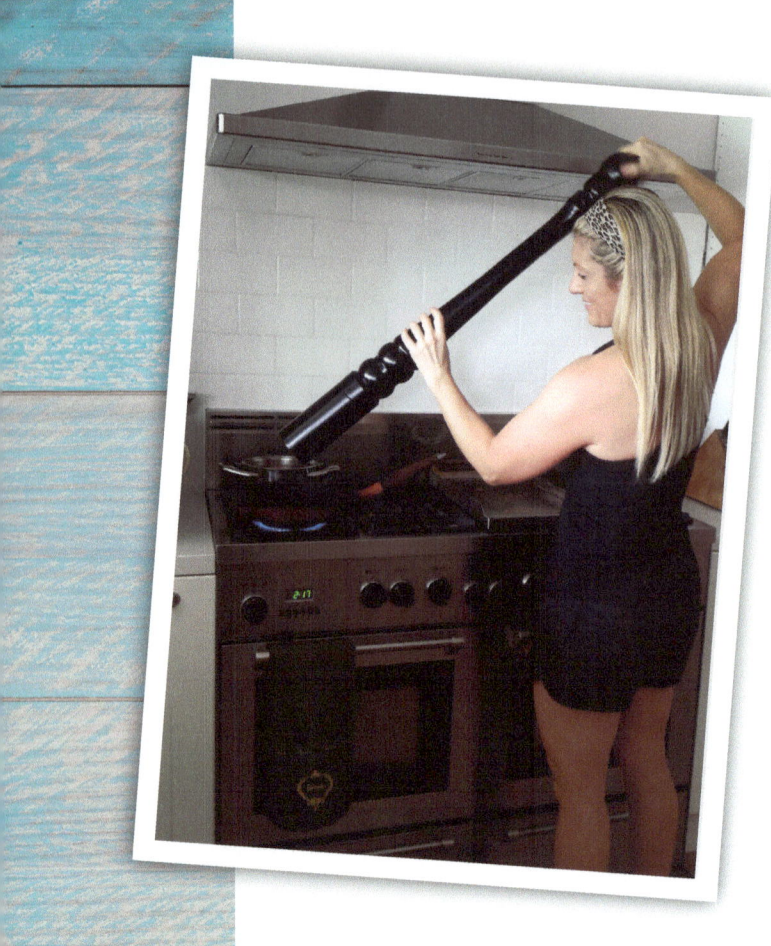

Helpful Tools for the Kitchen

Gadgets I can't live without and a few other useful tools!

A good, strong and powerful blender
Food processor
Non-stick sandwich press
Spiralizer (see page 91)
Cold-press juicer
Smoothie maker
Mini chopper (great for dips and sauces on the go, also great to use travelling)
My kitchen gadget graters
An assortment of round and square shaped cake tins in various sizes (preferably spring loaded) to assist with dessert creations

Steer away from starchy foods where possible

White rice, potatoes, white bread and flours, pasta etc. I use and eat a lot of sweet potato, yam and kumara as my alternatives to these otherwise starchy foods. This way I avoid feeling bloated, heavy or sluggish and have a much smoother functioning digestive system, and that for me is something to smile about!

Why I love to use a non-stick sandwich press for most of my cooking

Cooking with a non-stick sandwich press is so surprisingly easy and so convenient to use! You can walk away and do other things in the kitchen, knowing that your food is cooking away safely.

If you're anything like me and trying to prepare food with children around, it often feels next to impossible to cook.

A non-stick sandwich press is a safe way to cook food as it has a 'top' on it and wandering little fingers can't grab hot food, like they could with an open fry pan on the stove.

Using a sandwich press also means that you do not need to add any oil with your cooking (unless it's coconut oil of course) avoiding greasy food and oily pans to wash afterwards.

Why use pink Himalayan salt

Sea salt may dehydrate the body whereas Himalayan salt actually hydrates our tissue. Sea salt can be difficult to digest, whereas virtually no digestion is required for Himalayan salt. Not to mention, the taste of pink Himalayan salt is so much more alive and inviting.

Why cook with raw, cold pressed coconut oil

It is very resistant to oxidation at high heats, making it the perfect oil for cooking at high temperatures, especially using cooking methods such as frying. A lot of cooking oils can become toxic when heated past a certain point, but coconut oil does not. The unique taste that it infuses food with is absolutely delicious. It really is the oil of choice for a lifestyle of health.

Adore Nature's Milks

Making almond, nut and seed milks

Almond Milk

Soak a packet of raw almonds in water overnight (about 12 hours) to activate them. This brings out the full nutrient potential of the nut, and it also makes them easier to pulverize.

Rinse the nuts in a colander and then blend for several minutes until they are as smooth as possible. Add water or pure coconut milk as needed to make your milk even smoother and silkier.

Store in a sealed glass jar in the fridge. Activated almond milk (made with soaked almonds) will keep for around two to three days in a very cold fridge. Un-soaked almond milk will keep for up to five days.

You can get creative and add optional extras like; fresh vanilla pod, organic cinnamon and pure coconut water. You can also blend pitted medjool dates or add a dash of coconut syrup or raw honey through the mixture for a sweeter taste if using nut milk on something like morning oats.

You can use the same easy method to make your own milk with other nuts and seeds of choice.

I use this easy method to quickly whip up my own seed milk, like pepita milk and coconut milk varieties, as well as other varieties of nut milks like walnut.

Pepita and walnut milk is a delicious combination and worth a try!

In my pepita milk I also add a touch of organic turmeric powder with a tiny sprinkle of cracked pepper to activate the turmeric. This makes for an amazingly healthy 'milk' drink on its own, but you can also use it to pour over organic cereals, granola, rolled oats or use in smoothies.

Using a nut milk bag is another way to drain soaked blended nuts or seeds to get a smoother texture. The creative options are endless.

Coconut Milk – the milk of life

The regular fresh coconuts found at foodie markets and most fruit stores are great for making coconut milk.

Use two or three fresh coconuts, chop them in half over a large clean bowl, bucket or tub, to catch all the coconut water..

You will need to chop the coconut with a big knife or a small axe-like tool, taking the utmost care of course, or better still have your local coconut supplier assist you.

Scrape out the white coconut flesh with a sharp knife. You can do this by carefully making incisions in the coconut flesh first and then remove the flesh through the knife blade grip of the incisions so you are left with slices and pieces of fresh coconut.

Place the slices and pieces of the white flesh of the coconuts into a high-powered blender, along with the coconut water. Blend until thick, creamy milk is formed.

If you are after an even smoother texture, use a nut milk bag to drain the blended coconut mixture.

The health benefits, the taste, the smell. This milk truly is the milk of life!

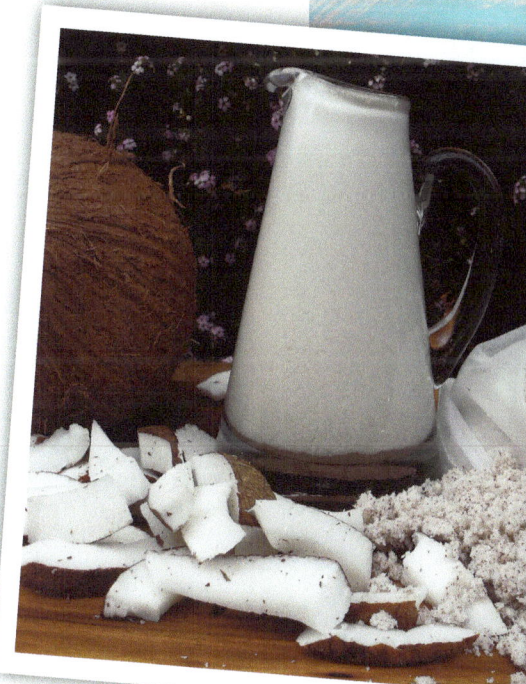

Create different and delicious coconut milk tastes by adding optional extras like; fresh vanilla pod, organic cinnamon, pure coconut water, blended pitted medjool dates or add a dash of coconut syrup through the mixture.

Make your own LSA

LSA (linseeds/sunflower seeds/almonds) is a super healthy raw nut and seed mix. It tastes great in shakes, smoothies, on morning oats, over salads or fruit salad, even sprinkled over pumpkin soup!

3 cups raw linseeds, flaxseeds or chia seeds
2 cups raw sunflower seeds
1 1/2 cups raw almonds

Grind all seeds and nuts in a food processor, until it becomes a fine meal
Store in a glass airtight jar or container in the fridge – it will last for up to 3 months.
I use LSA in my Morning Pow (see page22) and it tastes amazing!

Natural Alternative Protein Powders

These protein powders are all-natural, plant-based, organic, gluten free, dairy free, GMO free, and contain no additives or preservatives, no lactose or artificial sweeteners, no artificial colours or flavours, no pesticides or animal products. They are available at most organic and health food stores.

Natural plant-based protein powders are great alternatives to whey protein. Whey protein can cause bloating and/or stomach upset, and can often be harder to digest.

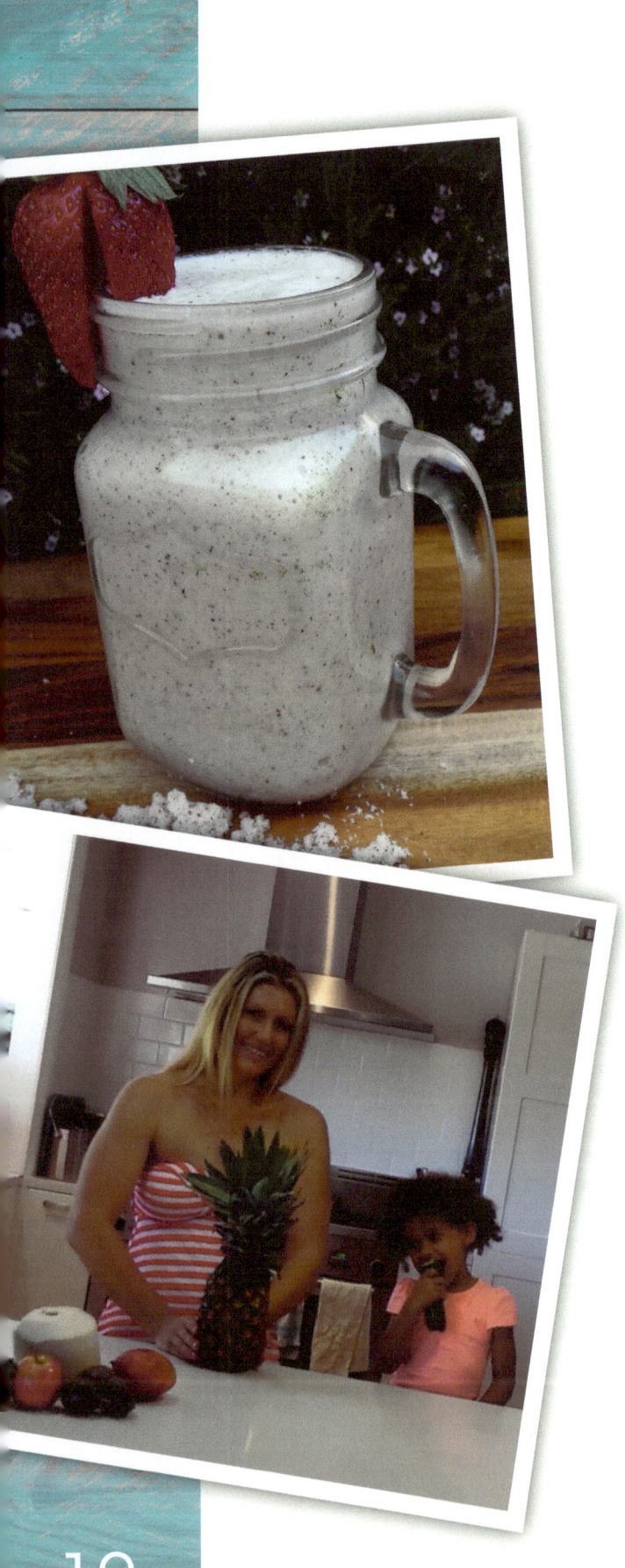

"I prefer plant-based proteins cause they are easier to digest."

Adore Juices and Smoothies

Cold Press Juices & Smoothies

Juices and smoothies are such a wonderful way to cleanse and revitalise your body. I juice on a daily basis. When juicing for a few days in a row, it gives your body a rest from the hard work of digesting solid food. It also works wonders for shedding unwanted pounds, plus it benefits your health in the long run. When in doubt, juice it out!

I buy a lot of fresh fruit to use in my juices and smoothies and I also use a fair amount of that organic fresh fruit to freeze. I don't buy packet frozen fruit – ever. Again, it is about knowing exactly where your produce has come from and that goes for frozen fruits as well.

TIP: I always keep and use my bananas that are looking over-ripe – they are at the ideal stage for getting best nutritional benefits. I peel them and freeze them. They really come in handy for whipping up a quick drink, smoothie, ice-cream, dessert, and all sorts of nutritious treats at any time!

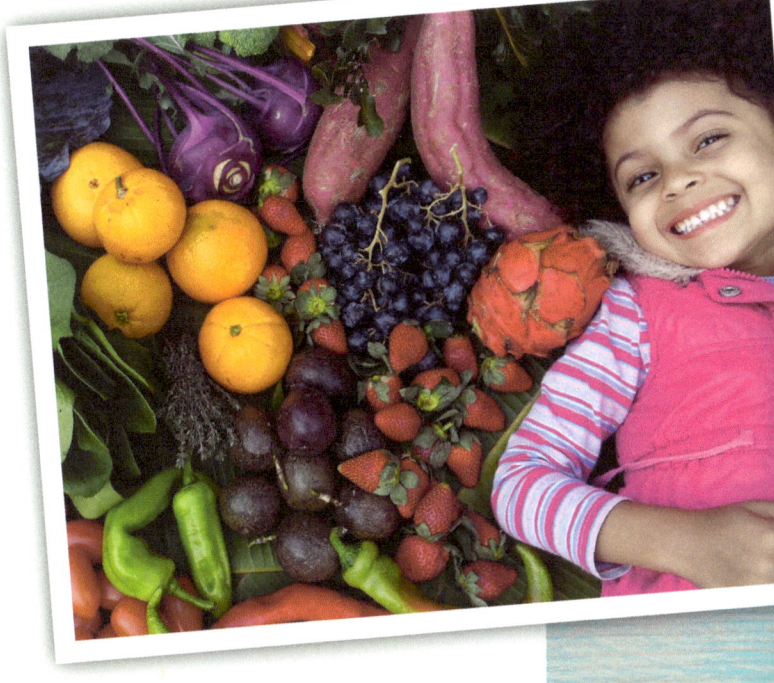

Directions for all juice recipies

Clean and wash all ingredients well. Then chop, slice and cut all fruits and vegetables to make cold-press juicing or blending easier. Some cold-press juicers allow the fruit and vegetables to be placed in whole which is ideal. Others have a narrow opening so cutting up fruits and vegetables may be needed. Juice all fruits and vegetables, especially oranges, limes and lemons, with their skins on (washed well of course) for obtaining maximum nutrients, fibre, minerals and vitamins, plus it makes for a better flavour!

Always make cold-pressed juice when juicing because it produces a healthier juice – all the vitamins and minerals are being used. Often regular juicing can strip some essential vitamins and minerals through the process. When juices are cold-pressed it helps keep the nutrients and enzymes intact and alive.

Cold-pressed juices are a great way for your body to get the maximum benefit from fruits and vegetables. It's about getting ALL the goodness into your body!

Important: All of my juices can be created using a blender, but make sure to add a good cup of purified water when blending.

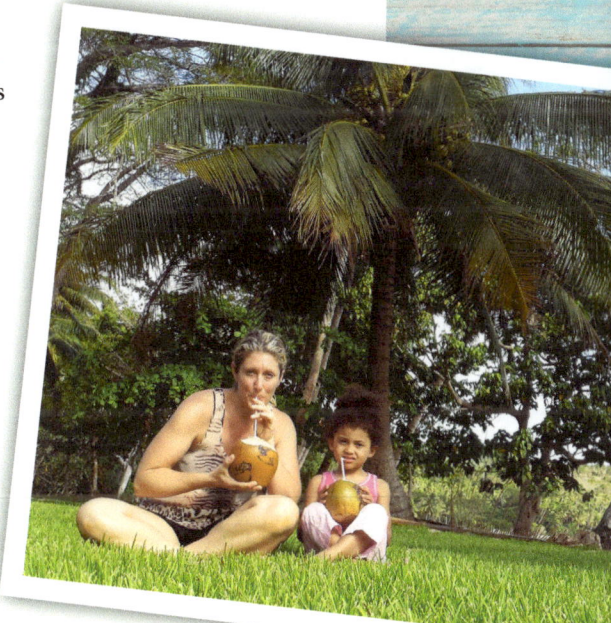

Smoothies

Tip: I use frozen fruits that I have already pre-prepared in my freezer. Making them as cold as possible makes the smoothie more enjoyable.

A daily recommendation: Drink wheat grass shots daily, and where possible include wheatgrass in your juices, because it's a superior detoxification agent. I simply love how this powerful component has the ability to slow down the aging process and it is an effective healer as it contains every mineral there possibly is! It is also a super rich source of protein. You can literally feel its goodness working through your system just minutes after drinking it. If you're finding it hard to get your energy levels back, a regular morning shot of wheatgrass will do that and more for you and your body. Wheatgrass can be a little bitter so I like to eat a strawberry straight after a wheatgrass shot, or I have a piece of fresh orange or something citrus.

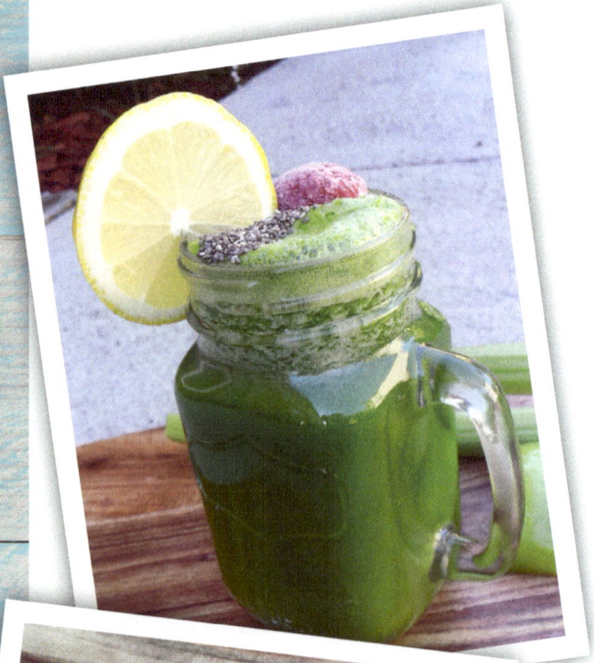

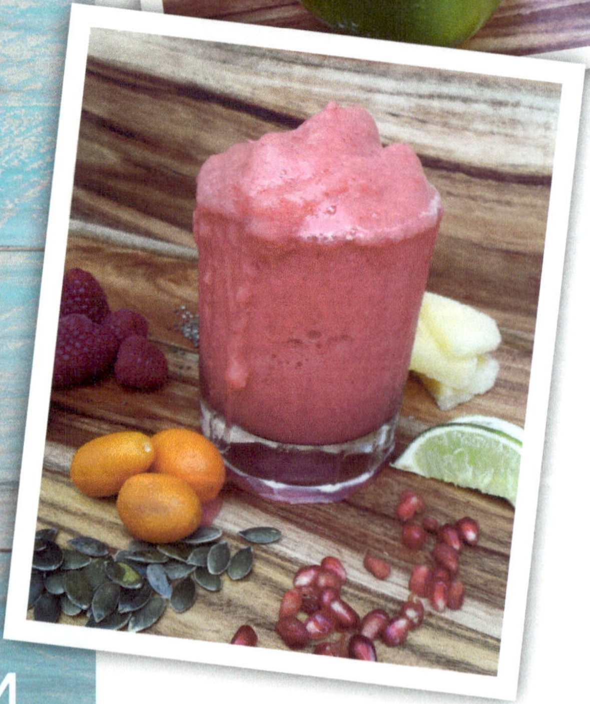

The Green Machine (pictured left)

2 green apples
2 celery stalks
8 Russian kale leaves
1 large lemon, cold pressed with skin on
1 thumb-sized piece of ginger

Antioxidant Booster

1 handful strawberries, stems removed
1/2 pineapple, skin removed
1 handful blueberries
1 handful raspberries
1 handful baby spinach leaves
1 handful of fresh mint, stalks and all
1 lime, washed with skin left on
1 tbsp of chia seeds
3/4 cup purified water if using a blender

Berry Bliss (pictured left)

Any fresh berries will work with this bliss drink, but this is what I really like to combine for my Berry Bliss experience.

1/2 punnet fresh or frozen strawberries
1/2 punnet fresh or frozen raspberries
Seeds of 1 pomegranate
1/2 red dragon fruit, skin removed
1 cup pure organic coconut cream (optional)

The coconut cream gives this drink a much creamier texture, but the fruit combined together on its own is also a pure delight to enjoy.

Nature's Pina Colada (pictured right)

1 ripe pineapple, skin removed
1 large handful fresh mint, stalks and all
1 handful of ice cubes
1 cup pure coconut water (I use direct from fresh real coconuts)

Fresh Breathe Juice

3 green apples
1 quarter watermelon, cold pressed with skin on
1 whole fennel bulb (stalks, leaves, seeds, bulbs and all)
1 handful fresh mint leaves

Midday Power Kick

1 ripe mango
1 large ripe banana (can be frozen)
1/2 tsp of nutmeg
1 tbsp chia seeds
1 large handful fresh raspberries

The Carrot Kiss - eyesight and brain function improver (pictured right)

5 - 6 large organic carrots
1 large thumb-sized piece of fresh ginger
1 large thumb-sized piece of fresh turmeric
1/2 tsp cracked black pepper (I use cracked black pepper to activate the turmeric)

The Calmer (pictured right)

3 large chilled red ruby grapefruit, cold pressed with skin on
1 large handful ice cubes
1 handful fresh mint leaves (optional)

*add a drop of grapefruit 100% pure essential oil for an extra health boost

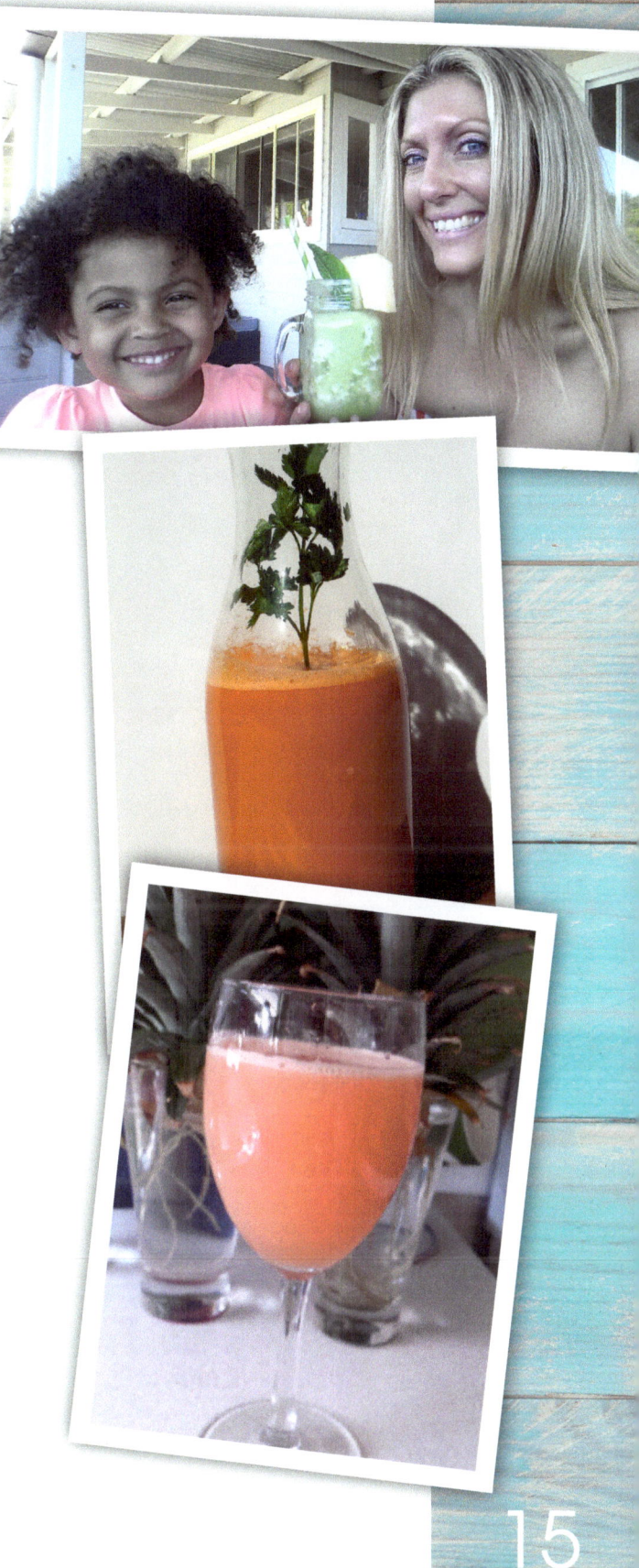

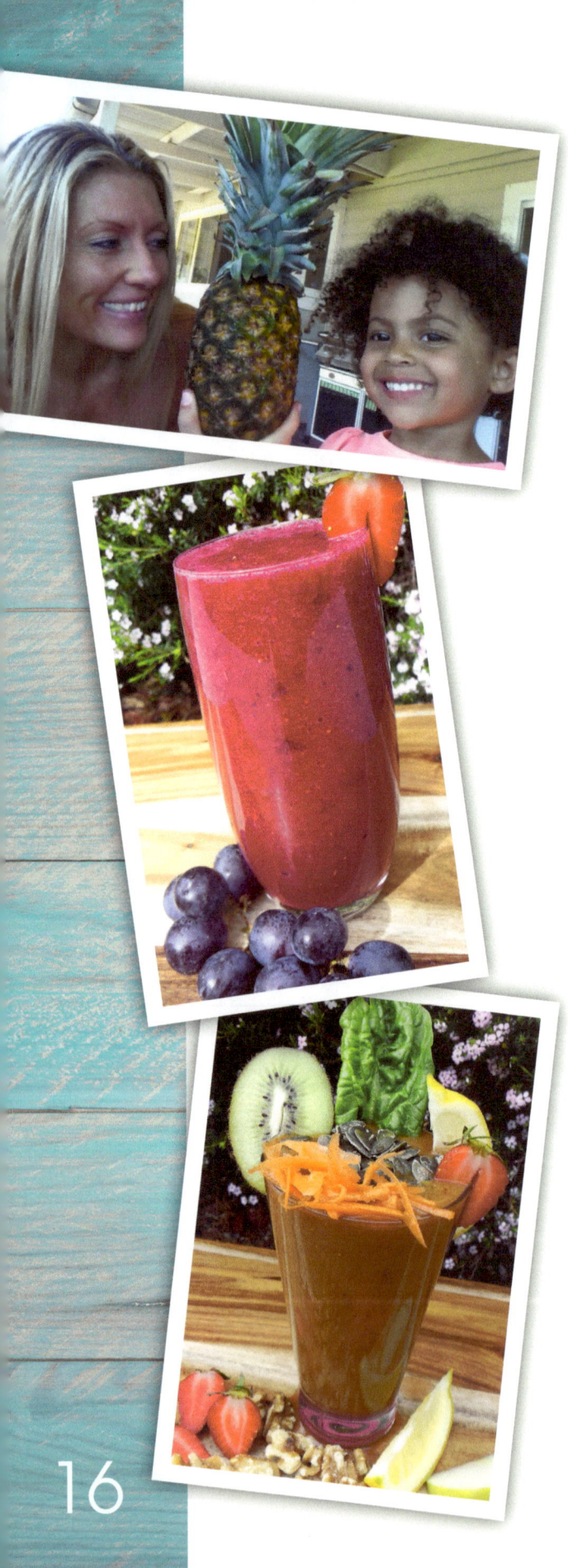

Pineapple, Lemon, Ginger Juice

1 whole pineapple, skin removed

1 large fresh lemon, washed and skin kept on
1 thumb-sized piece of ginger, washed and skin on

I drink this juice when I have a cold or cough. Pineapple juice does wonders!

Red Divine (pictured left)

1 fresh red beetroot , skin kept on
1 punnet strawberries, stalks removed
1 large bunch dark red grapes

1 thumb-sized piece of fresh ginger
3/4 cup purified water if blending

Handy tip: did you know loading up on organic strawberries before exercising can give you greater endurance and even burn more calories?

Handy tip: did you know eating dark red organic grapes can play a protective role in avoiding many illnesses and diseases, as well as viral and fungal infections?

Skin Glow and Repair Juice (pictured left)

2 ripe kiwifruit
2 green apples
1 lemon, washed and skin on
1 handful pepitas
1 carrot
1/2 punnet strawberries, stems removed
1 handful baby spinach
1 handful walnuts
4 fresh apricots (when in season), stones removed

Make your impossible a reality. Bring extraordinary every day. Believe.

Immune Defence Shot (pictured right)

2 limes, with skin kept on
1 large thumb-sized piece of fresh ginger
1 tsp cayenne pepper
1 lemon, with skin kept on
1 large thumb-sized piece of fresh turmeric
1 orange, with skin kept on
1 medium-sized red chilli, remove stem

Daily Energizer

3 large carrots
1 red beetroot, skin on
3 celery stalks
1 thumb-sized piece of fresh ginger
4 kale leaves with stems
1 large handful Italian parsley

Avocado Smoothie (pictured right)

1 ripe avocado, seed and skin removed
2 frozen bananas
1 cup coconut water direct from the coconut
1 cup fresh coconut flesh, from the same fresh coconut
1/2 cup ice
Blend well together till thick and creamy.

Note: add 1/2 cup raw organic cacao powder to turn this into a delicious healthy chocolate smoothie

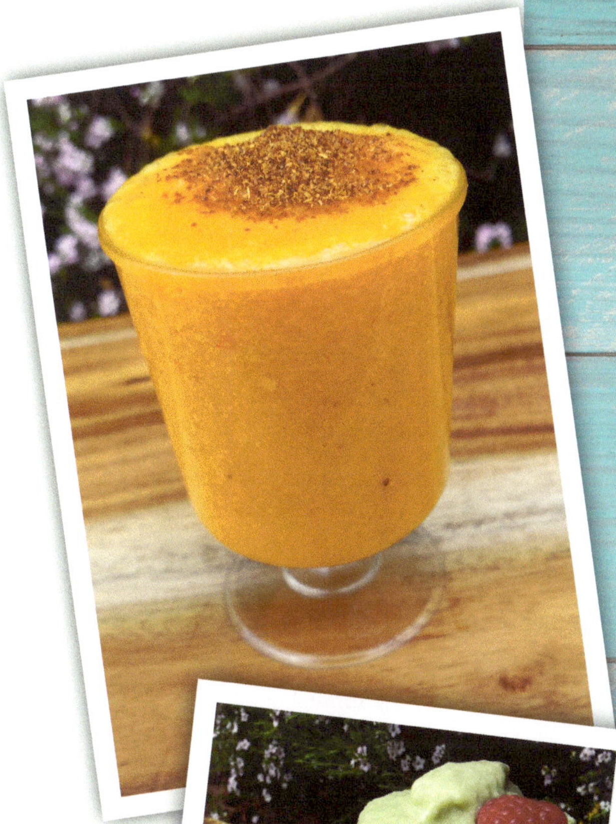

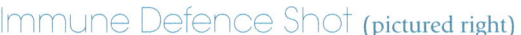
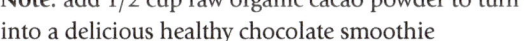

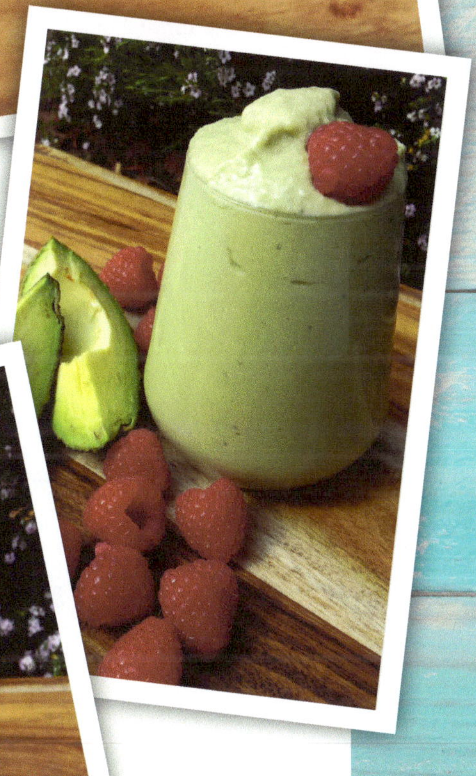

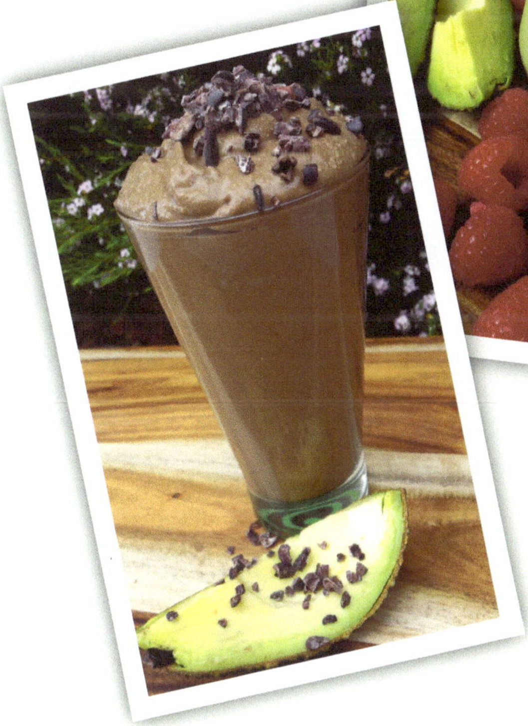

Adore Mornings

Eggs and Omelettes

Eggs and omelettes can be enjoyed in so many delicious styles.

If you choose to eat eggs, make sure you know exactly where they have come from. I believe it is important not to contribute to the cruelty of factory farming.

'Organic' and 'free range' does not necessarily exclude factory-farming cruelty.

If I eat eggs, I get them direct from friends or family who have chickens in their back yards, roaming free. That way I know exactly what I'm eating and exactly where it's come from.

I suggest that where possible, eggs need to be biodynamic and from chickens that are pasture raised, cruelty free (no beak trimming or other abuse), chemical free, pesticide free, GMO free, herbicide free, open freely ranging at the free range standard of no more than the maximum number of specified birds allowed per hectare.

If you're not choosing to eat eggs, scrambled or fried tofu (cooked in coconut oil) is a great alternative.

Morning is a great time to eat good carbohydrates and good fats. Eating good fats in the morning will give you energy throughout the day and assist with burning unwanted body fat. Avocado is a great source of good fats and, coupled with sweet potato, provides fuel and energy for the body to burn. I love a sweet potato of a morning, with some delicious ripe avocado!

Here are some of the many different ways to enjoy eating eggs and omelettes…

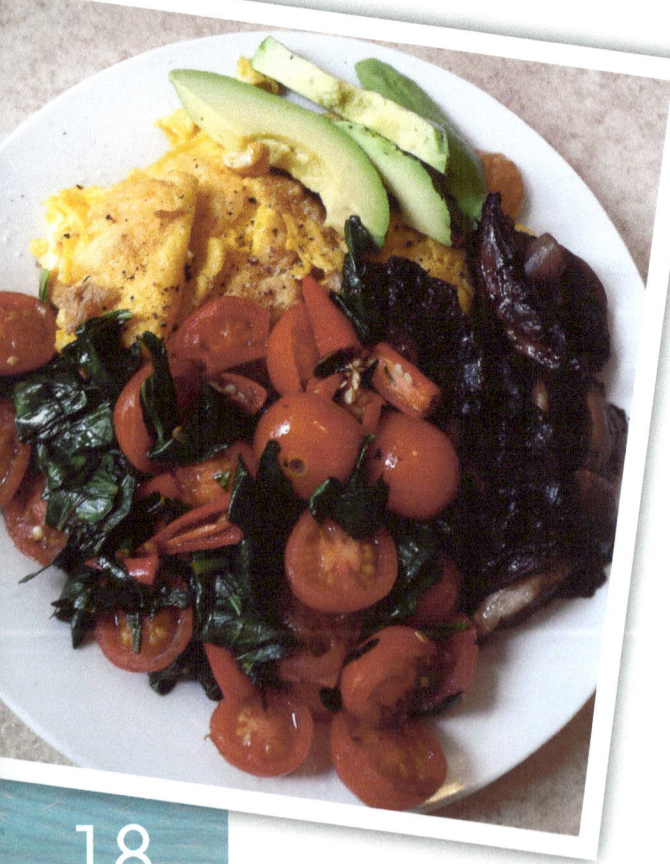

Folded Egg with Fresh Basil, Chilli and Cherry tomato stir-fry, Coconut fried mushrooms and cooling avocado

3 eggs, whisked together
1/2 punnet of cherry tomatoes, cut into halves
3 fresh red chillies, chopped into pieces with stems removed
1 large handful fresh basil, roughly chopped
250g mushrooms of choice, roughly chopped
1/2 ripe avocado
Himalayan pink salt and cracked black pepper

Cook the eggs until golden brown in a small fry pan with 1 tablespoon of coconut oil. When done, fold in half and place on serving plate.
In the same pan, stir-fry your tomatoes and chilli. When done, add to the side of the plate next to the eggs.
In the same fry pan, and with another tablespoon of coconut oil, cook the mushrooms.
Place this onto your plate, sprinkle everything with the basil, salt and pepper.

This is one of my favourite ways to eat eggs – so enjoy! To make the above recipe into an 'English Spinach Scrambled Egg Medley', try a large handful of English spinach and slices of avocado to serve with.

Warm Egg Salad (pictured right)

2 eggs scrambled in coconut oil with a sprinkle of pink Himalayan salt and cracked black pepper
1/2 ripe avocado, scooped out into pieces
1 dollop of organic Greek yoghurt
1/2 cucumber, chopped
1/4 sweet potato, cut into pieces and cooked in non-stick sandwich press
5 grape tomatoes, halved

Place all ingredients onto serving plate and garnish with coriander. Enjoy!

Kale and Feta Omelette

Heat a small, non-stick frying pan, adding 1 tablespoon of coconut oil.
Whisk 3 eggs and add to the pan.

Add:
1/2 bunch Russian kale or spinach, chopped
10 whole cherry tomatoes
50g goats cheese, cut into pieces and sprinkled over the top
1 pinch each of Himalayan salt and cracked black pepper over cooking ingredients

Cook through until all ingredients are done.
Turn out from the pan onto a serving plate and enjoy!

Easy Omelette - sandwich press style

This style of omelette cooking is fantastic because it's more than just easy. It leaves next to no mess to clean up and it literally only takes a few minutes to complete.
Place a thumb-sized amount of coconut oil onto non-stick sandwich press while it is heating.
Crack 3 eggs into a small bowl and whisk together. Pour the eggs onto heated sandwich press.
Place English spinach and whole cherry or grape tomatoes on top of the eggs and close the sandwich press allowing to cook for two to three minutes.
Fold egg over the spinach and tomatoes from the sides ensuring the whole omelette is cooked through.
Place onto a serving plate and garnish with sprinkle of pink Himalayan salt, cracked black pepper and fresh herbs. Enjoy!

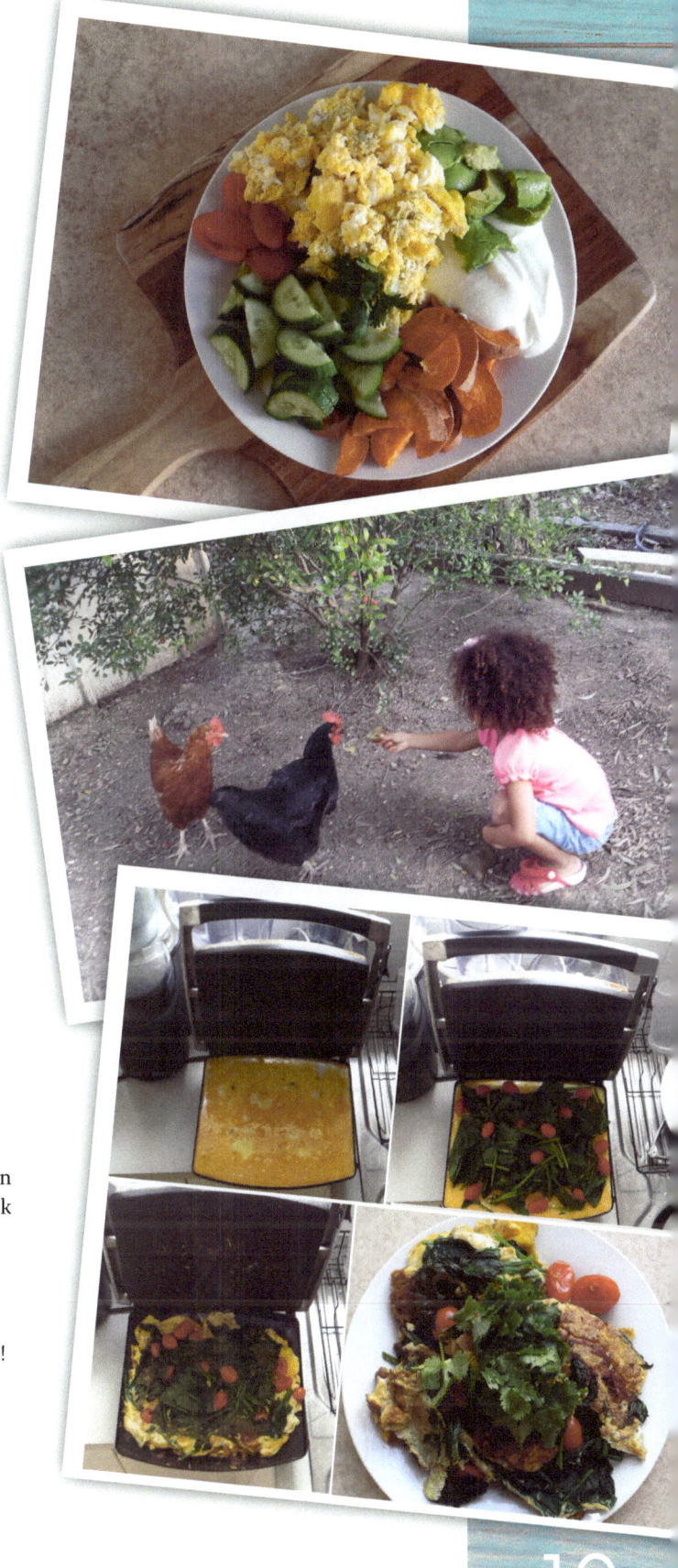

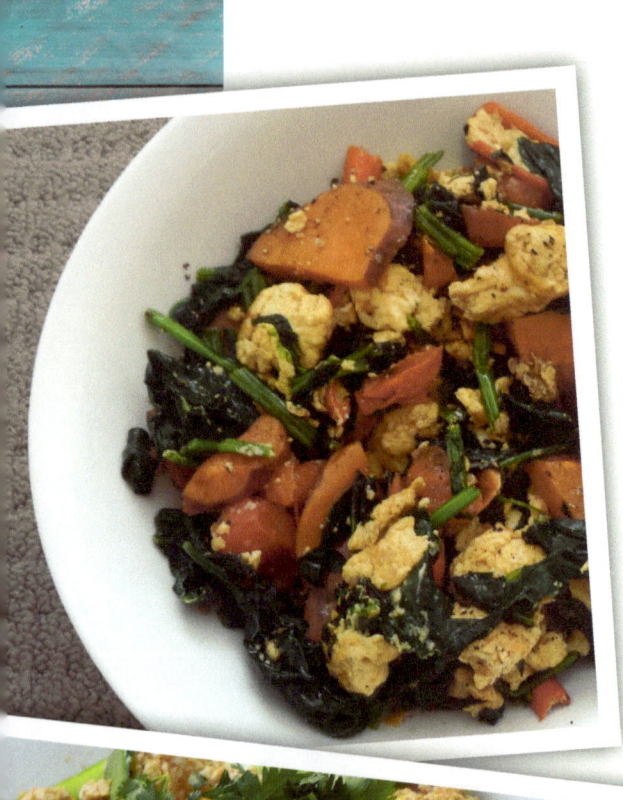

Egg and Vege Fry Up

This is a great morning energy booster that will keep your system going for the entire day!

1/2 sweet potato, chopped into pieces and cooked on a non-stick sandwich press
3 eggs
1/2 punnet cherry tomatoes, halved
1 large handful of english spinach
1/4 head of broccoli
2 red chillies, stems removed and chopped

In a non-stick frying pan place 1 heaped tablespoon of coconut oil. Crack the eggs into the pan and whisk over the heat, adding the cherry tomatoes.
Add the spinach, broccoli and chilli and continue to cook.
Lastly add the cooked sweet potato into the pan, with a sprinkle of Himalayan salt and cracked black pepper, and a drizzle of fresh lemon juice.
Turn out onto serving plate and enjoy the delicious goodness.

Bok Choy, Fresh Chilli, Herb and Kumara Eggs

This is definitely up there on my list of favourite ways to eat eggs and a real system 'fire up' to start the day.

2 eggs, whisked
1 bunch fresh bok choy, separated and washed
2 red chilli, chopped with stems removed
1/2 kumara, cut into medium thick slices
1 bunch fresh coriander, chopped
1 large handful fresh Italian parsley, chopped
1 tbsp raw and cold pressed coconut oil

Cook the kumara in a non-stick sandwich press, or frying pan, until soft and golden.
In a hot pan with 1 tablespoon of coconut oil, add the eggs and cook till fluffy and golden.
Add the bok choy, chilli and cooked kumara into the hot pan, combining all ingredients.
Place onto a serving plate, season with Himalayan salt and cracked black pepper, garnish with coriander and Italian parsley.

Create a greater you with every day, for with every day there is great opportunity.

A healthy life starts with healthy thoughts.

Morning meal time

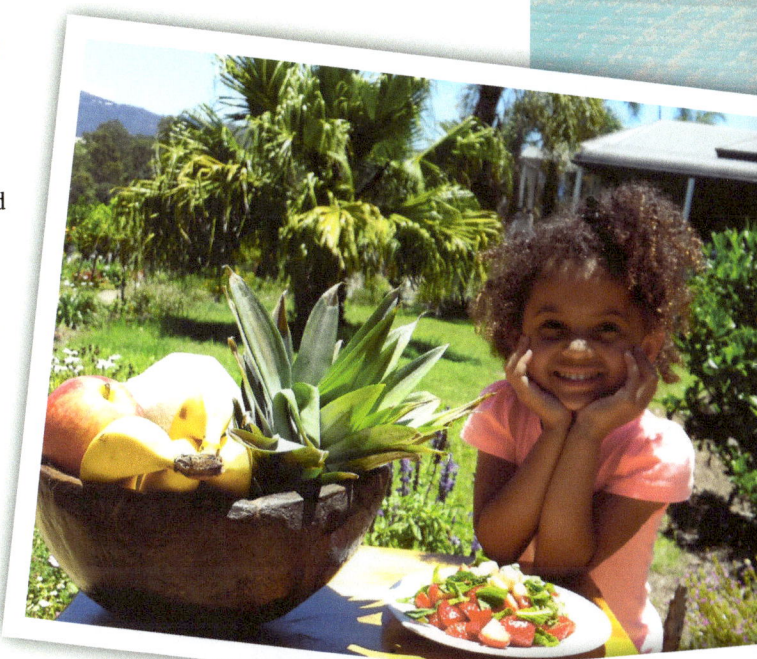

As we have all heard over the years, breakfast is the most important meal of the day, and it's true! Your body won't perform and work to its best ability if it hasn't been fuelled correctly. Breakfast has got to be one of my favourite meal times. There's something exciting about waking up in the morning and eating to energise yourself for the day. These are some of my favourite nourishing and healthy morning meal options to help kick-start the day in the right way!

Avocado Muesli

There are so many delicious ways to create muesli, but this is one way that I like to make, eat and enjoy it.

3/4 cup raw almonds
3/4 cup raw macadamias
3/4 cup raw hazelnuts
2 cups coconut flakes
2 tbsp sesame seeds
1 heaped tbsp coconut sugar
2 tsp organic cinnamon
1 ripe avocado
1 handful fresh blueberries
1/2 punnet fresh strawberries, tops removed and cut into quarters

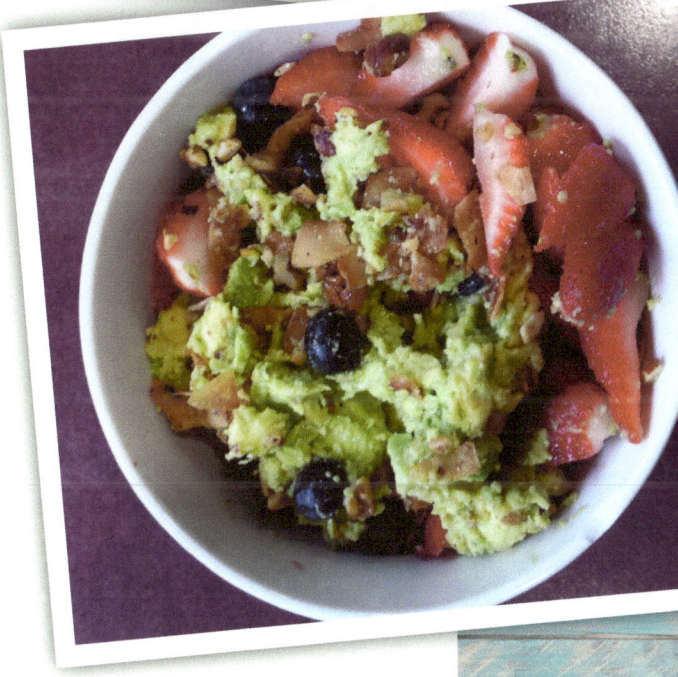

This can be eaten as it is by mixing all the dry ingredients together, then mashing the avocado through with a garnish of blueberries and strawberries, or it can also be roasted.
To Roast: pre-heat oven to 200 degrees. Place almonds, macadamias and hazelnuts on a baking tray and cook for seven minutes taking care not to let them burn. Add coconut flakes, sesame seeds and coconut sugar to the tray, stirring through, and cook for a further three minutes, again keeping a close eye on the tray.
Place on cooling tray. When the muesli mixture has cooled, sprinkle over cinnamon, stir through then place desired amount in serving bowl. Mash ripe avocado with a fork in a separate bowl then add to roasted muesli. Garnish with blueberries and strawberries and enjoy!

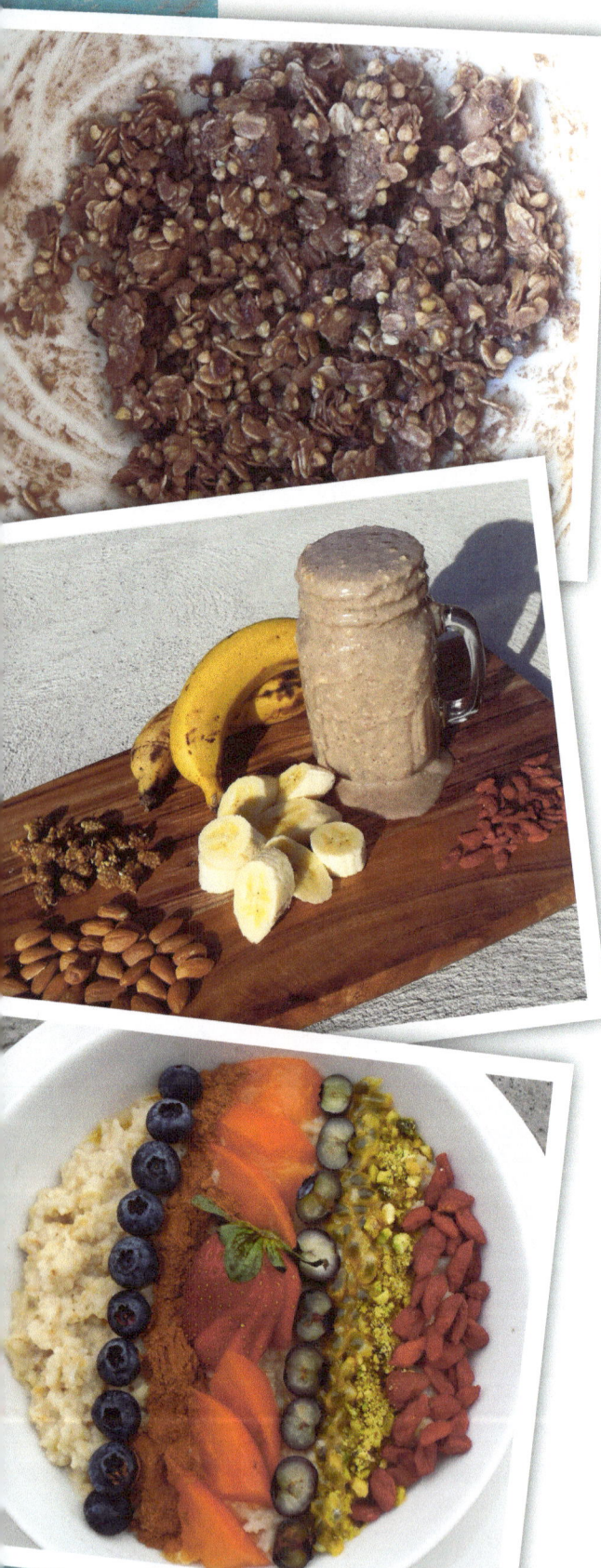

Raw Choc Granola

Just the sound of this dish seems so naughty, but this delicious raw granola is far from that – it's a guilt-free morning energy booster with scrumptious flavour. Super easy to make, it is a 'get up and go' kind of breakfast.

1 cup organic activated plain Buckinis
2 tbsp raw cacao nibs
1 cup organic coconut flakes
1/2 cup raw organic cacao powder
1 cup organic rolled oats (gluten free option: quinoa flakes)
5 pitted medjool dates, finely chopped
1 heaped tbsp coconut oil, melted to liquid state
1 generous sprinkle organic cinnamon
1 scoop chocolate plant-based protein powder
1 pinch Himalayan salt
1 handful raw macadamias or almonds, crushed

Mix all ingredients together. Eat with fresh slices of banana, kiwifruit or strawberries. Also tastes great with a dash of almond milk. Enjoy!

Morning POW

I absolutely adore this morning 'pow' drink. Every time I have this, my energy levels jump and I really feel fired up for the day.

2 large frozen bananas
2 tbsp of organic LSA mix (linseeds, sunflower seeds and almonds, see page 12)
1 handful of raw almonds (preferably activated)
1 tbsp organic cinnamon
2 cups organic almond milk (see page 11 for almond milk recipe) or water will do just fine if no almond milk on hand
1 scoop plant-based chocolate protein powder

Blend all ingredients together well and enjoy!

Morning Rainbow Oats

Soak 1 cup of raw organic rolled oats in water overnight (soaking oats makes them easier for your system to digest).
Cook the soaked oats for two to four minutes on a high heat, with an extra 1/2 cup of water.
Place into breakfast serving bowl.
Add toppings such as fresh blueberries, organic cinnamon, persimmon, strawberries, passionfruit, raw pistachios and goji berries.
These oats are delicious to eat on their own with the toppings, or you can add a dash of almond or nut milk (see page 11 for milk) with a drizzle of raw honey.

Blueberry Pancakes

This makes for an awesome and healthy morning treat. I can't resist these delicious homemade pancakes.

2 1/2 cups almond meal
1 dash of almond milk or purified water
1/2 cup coconut oil, melted to liquid form
1 1/2 punnets fresh blueberries
1 very ripe banana
1/2 cup almond flakes or crushed almonds to decorate
1 drizzle coconut syrup or sprinkle of organic cinnamon to decorate
1 dollop of organic Greek yoghurt (optional)
1 banana, cut into slices to decorate

Blend ripe banana with 1 punnet of blueberries and dash of purified water or almond milk.
Combine almond meal and 3/4 of the liquid coconut oil in a bowl and mix together.
Add the blended banana and blueberry mixture to the bowl.
Heat the remaining coconut oil in a small non-stick pan or sandwich press.
Pour pancake-sized amounts of the batter into the heated pan or press.
Cook pancakes until golden brown both sides. When cooked, place on a serving board with slices of banana between each pancake as they are stacked.
Decorate with the remaining fresh blueberries, crushed almonds or almond flakes, a delicious drizzle of coconut syrup and a dollop of organic Greek yoghurt if desired.
These pancakes are so moist and inviting! Enjoy!

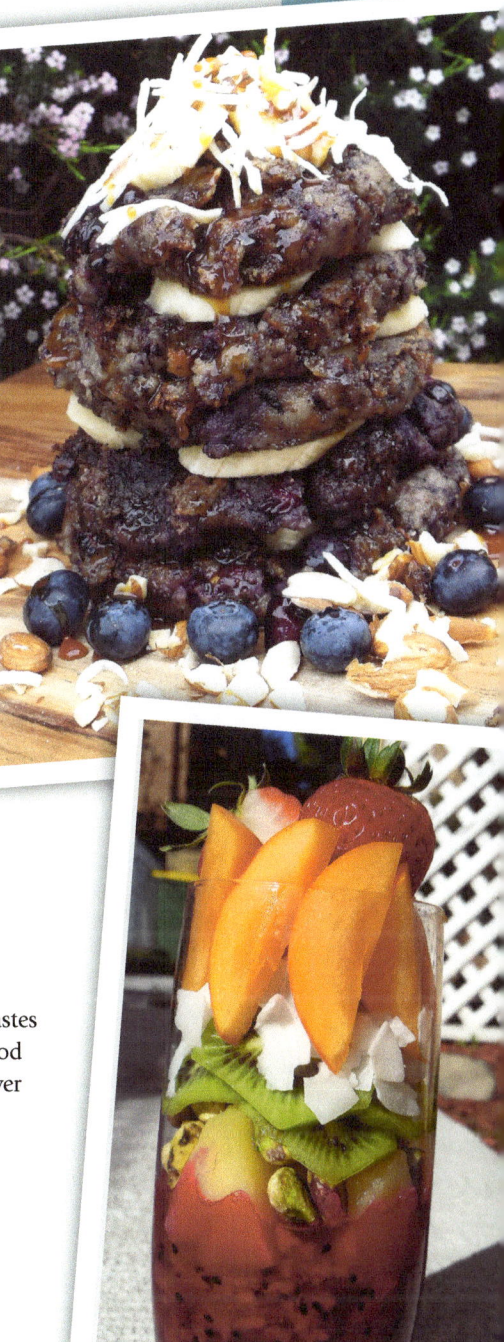

Layered Tropical fruits with pistachio nibs

Exotic tropical fruits are pieces of nature. I am not only inspired by the incredible tastes and colours, but also the natural goodness that comes from these fruits. There is good reason nature provides us with the foods it does. Try this refreshing tropical fruit layer to awaken your senses and energise you.

1/2 fresh red dragonfruit
1 slice fresh pineapple, skin removed, cut into small triangles
1 handful pistachio nibs
1 kiwifruit, cut into slices
1 handful organic coconut flakes
1 persimmon, cut in half then sliced
1 strawberry, cut in half

Scoop out the flesh from the dragonfruit into a small bowl and press with fork to smooth out.
Gently place the dragonfruit in the bottom of serving glass.
Place fresh pineapple pieces on top, standing into the dragonfruit with the points facing upward.
Sprinkle with pistachio nibs, layer in some kiwifruit pieces, sprinkle on some coconut flakes and place sliced persimmon in upright positions around top of glass.
Place the two strawberry halves, point down, in the centre. Enjoy!

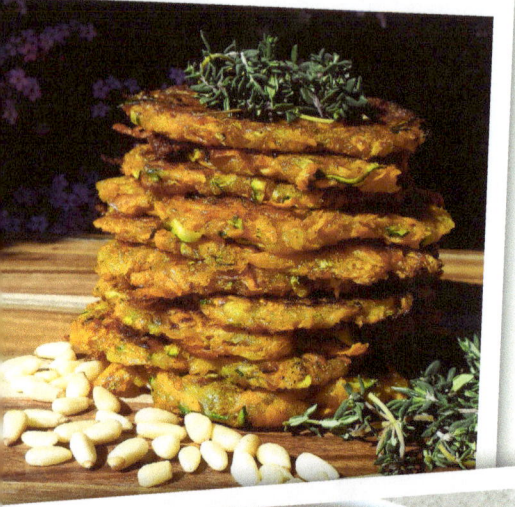

Easy Savoury Pancakes

Yes, savoury pancakes for your morning meal! I eat sweet potato because it's a good carbohydrate to have in the morning, it gives me energy to burn throughout the day and these taste so good and only require four ingredients to make.

1 large sweet potato, grated
2 medium-sized zucchinis, grated
1 cup psyllium husk
6 tbsp raw and cold pressed coconut oil, melted

Mix all ingredients together well. With clean hands create pancake 'patties' (about palm-sized) and place in a hot non-stick sandwich press. Cook till golden brown on both sides. Stack pancakes and garnish with fresh herbs.

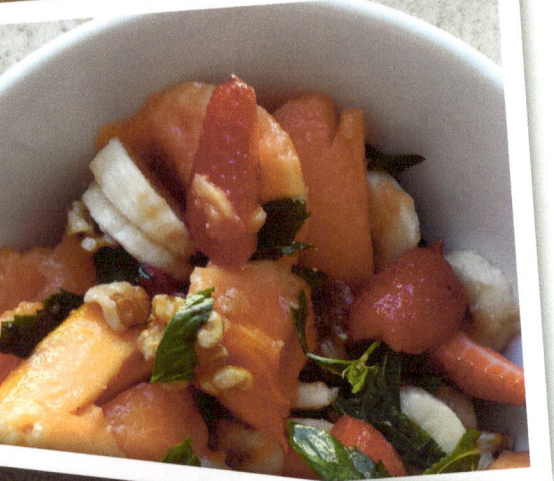

Paw Paw and Fresh Mint Fruit Salad

Such a refreshing morning pick me up! Fruit salad in the morning can awaken all the senses.

For my paw paw fruit salad creation you will need:
1 small paw paw, cut into small pieces with seeds removed (don't throw seeds away... see page 77 for benefits of paw paw seeds)
1 ripe banana, sliced
1/2 punnet fresh strawberries, cut into small pieces
1 handful raw walnuts
1 handful raw macadamia nuts
1 handful fresh mint, chopped

Combine all ingredients in a serving bowl and enjoy!

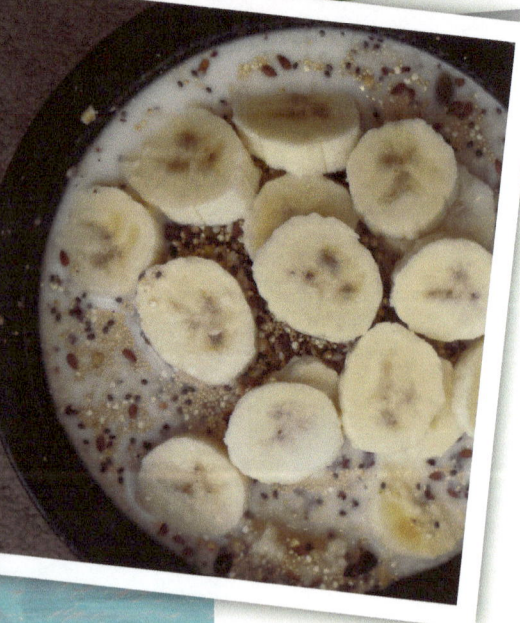

Banana, Nut Milk and Morning Seed Medley

I make up this seed mix and keep it sealed in an airtight container to have on hand. It goes well with rolled oats, in smoothies, sprinkled over cold-press juices, or simply on its own with homemade almond milk or a nut milk of my choice (see page 11) and freshly sliced banana. It's delicious!

All you need to do is combine:
1/2 cup of each of the following
flax seeds
Chia seeds
Pepita seeds
Organic activated plain Buckinis
Millet seeds
Linseed
Amaranth
Sunflower seeds
Sesame seeds

Mix together and keep in a sealed container. Enjoy with sliced banana and almond or nut milk or even a drizzle of raw honey.

Smashed Avocado and Jacket Kumara

This is a very satisfying morning meal and I often eat this. I usually prepare the jacket sweet potato or kumara the night before and reheat it in my non-stick sandwich press just before I'm about to eat it. This combination tastes so good and is so simple to put together.

1 jacket sweet potato or kumara, sliced in half horizontally and cooked at 180 degrees in the oven or non-stick sandwich press until soft on the inside but crisp on the outside. Place on serving board.
1 ripe avocado, smashed and mashed in a bowl with a squeeze of fresh lemon and a pinch of pink Himalayan salt (see page 49 for smashed avocado recipe). Smother over the kumara halves.
Crumble 100g goats cheese over the avocado.
Sprinkle 1 handful of finely shredded parsley on top of the goats cheese.
Season with Himalayan salt and cracked black pepper to taste, and sprinkle with 1/2 a cup of roasted pepitas.

As an option, I also like to drizzle it with a squeeze of fresh lemon or lime juice and add some freshly chopped chilli to spice things up.

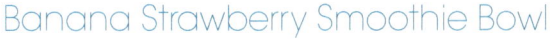

Banana Strawberry Smoothie Bowl

This is so delicious and one of my favourites, especially in the summer. The creamy banana flavour mixed with delicious sweet strawberries tastes divine. A nourishing, guilt-free start to the day.

2 frozen bananas
1 large handful frozen strawberries

Blend the fruit until smooth, thick and creamy.
Pour into a serving bowl and decorate with fresh fruit, nuts and seeds of your choice.
Enjoy!

Note: You can add which ever fresh, fruity flavours you prefer to this blend, popping them in during the blending process.

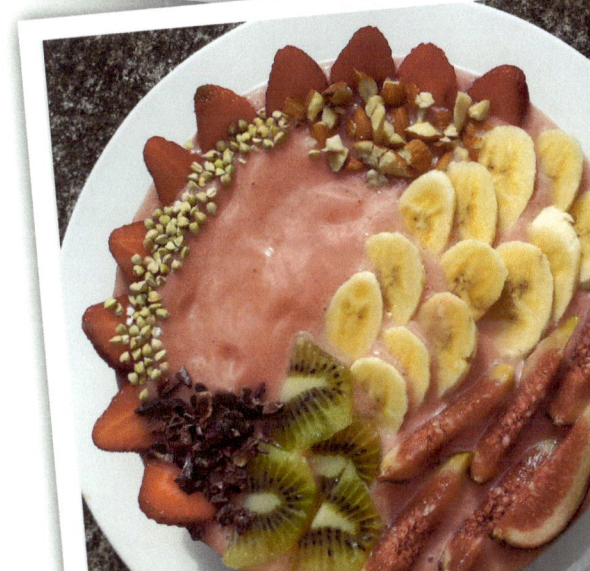

It doesn't matter how you arrive at your destination, just don't lose sight of the goal – stay focused and believe.

Adore Main Meals

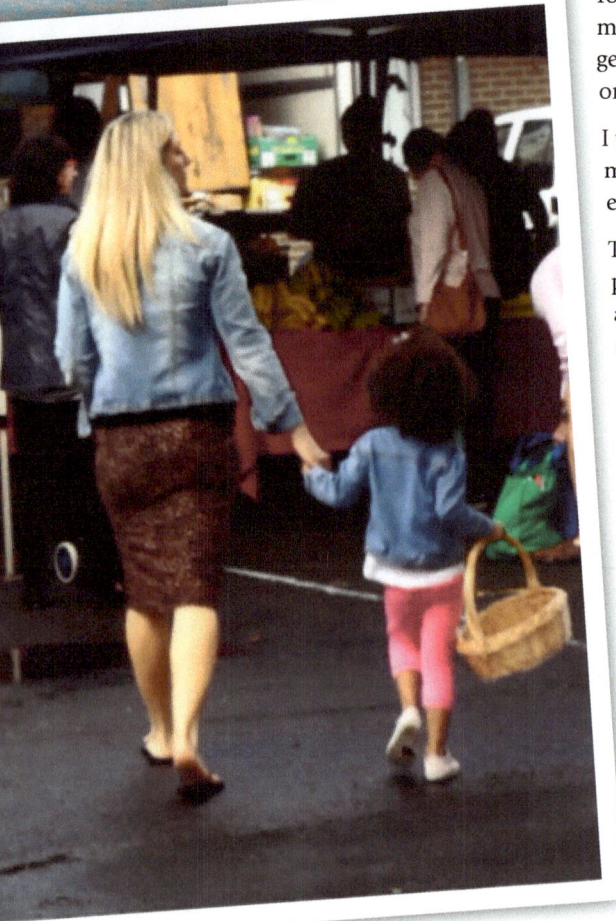

You don't really need much to create nourishing food and delicious meals – a little bit of imagination is all it takes! Thinking outside the box, getting those creative juices flowing ensures that the ingredients you have on hand can easily be transformed into delicious, healthy meals.

I tend to eat my main meal during the middle of the day to benefit my body as much as possible. I also use fresh chilli on anything and everything I can, as it is a fat burning favourite of mine.

Try and steer clear of eating anything from a can or packet where at all possible – the freshest most natural state is the best. I actually 'cook' as little as possible – the more raw food the better, as it's healthier and actually aids in fat loss.

With my food preparation, I always end up making twice as much food, which is probably force of habit from when I was growing up. It has turned out to be a handy trait. Now I am not actually cooking everyday. I have created my recipes and their sizes with this in mind. I have found its better to make more (and have the next few meals covered) than to make less.

I use a lot of simple herbs, oils and spices to create flavour in my food. The basics are often all you need. A simple lemon can impart such depth to a meal; Himalayan salt and cracked black pepper are a perfect way to make a meal complete. This is often what you will find me cooking with, aside from a few other fancy herbs or spices that can be added when appropriate. Creating dishes using fresh herbs and spices is the best way to get maximum nutrition, goodness and flavour, without any additives or preservatives. Often health problems that build up over time have been affected by our daily diet. Fresh herbs are a safe and satisfying way of eating, living and adoring a healthy lifestyle!

Raw plant-based whole foods

I love eating raw plant-based whole foods. Most of my meals are an introduction to this eating lifestyle and demonstrate how easy and tasty living a raw plant-based lifestyle can be, but all my meals can easily be catered to the cook's own personal tastes, eating styles and preferences. It's simply a matter of adding or removing ingredients. I have a huge love for nature and animals. For the most of my childhood I couldn't bear the thought of harming or killing animals, let alone eating them. I avoid eating meat mostly. However, you will find I have included meat in a few of my recipes - with vegetarian options.

For some time now I have been looking deeper into raw plant-based diets and how incredible the health benefits and quality of life are from eating in such a way. I am excited about the health advantages and natural healing properties for living a plant-based lifestyle. Adore Your Lifestyle has been a long time in the making, and taking this journey has revealed many deeper insights. I am always learning and discovering and look forward to scaling new health and nutritional heights, embarking on an even more exciting path in my health journey. All this through discovering raw food and plant-based eating options!

Raw Shaved Savoy and Zucchini noodles with Fresh Garlic Herb Sauce, Crispy Yam and Okra

This recipe is made using the tastes of Africa. Okra and yam are popular nutritious foods that I enjoyed during my time spent in South and West Africa. I have created this dish with the memories of those remarkable tastes, and added a sprinkle of Aussie flavour too!

1/2 savoy cabbage, finely chopped
3 medium zucchini, spiralized
1 large yam, washed and chopped into thick slices, then cooked until crispy and golden in a non-stick sandwich press
350g fresh okra, washed and kept whole, then cooked until crispy and golden in a non-stick sandwich press
Pinch of Himalayan salt

Place the spiralized zucchinis into a large bowl. Add finely diced savoy cabbage to the bowl, gently mixing together. Then add the sauce.
Sauce: (see garlic sauce page 48) blend all ingredients of the garlic sauce together, adding your choice of fresh herbs, until smooth (or leave slightly chunky if preferred) pour sauce over the savoy cabbage and zucchini noodles and mix through well.
Place in the centre of a large serving dish. Add cooked yam pieces and okra around the serving dish, sprinkle over some Himalayan salt and enjoy!
Optional and quick alternative: using only zucchini, cabbage and fresh herbs with your choice of freshly made sauce.

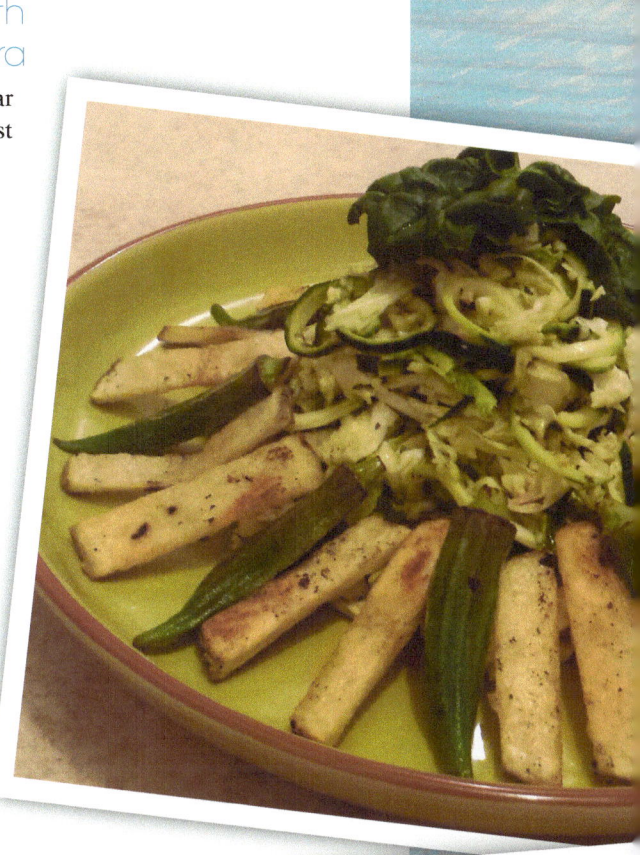

Avocado Rice Salad

This is such a fun, tasty and simple dish to put together. I make a large amount and store it for a day or so in the fridge – it makes for a great dish to have on the run, both hot or cold.

1 cup good quality organic brown or black rice, boiled (you can use 1 shredded cauliflower cooked up in coconut oil as a rice alternative – it tastes amazing)
2 large ripe avocados, mashed with the juice of 1 lemon
1 carrot, finely diced
1 purple onion, finely diced
1 punnet cherry or grape tomatoes, diced (I like to use orange and yellow tomatoes for more vibrant colour in the meal)
1 bunch fresh coriander, finely chopped
1 handful fresh snow peas for garnish

In a large bowl add carrot, tomatoes, onion, chopped coriander and rice. Stir together.
Add mashed avocado and evenly mix throughout the rice. Place on serving plate. Add coriander and snowpeas on top for garnish. Enjoy! This recipe can also be enjoyed with hot corn on the cob or fresh grilled fish.

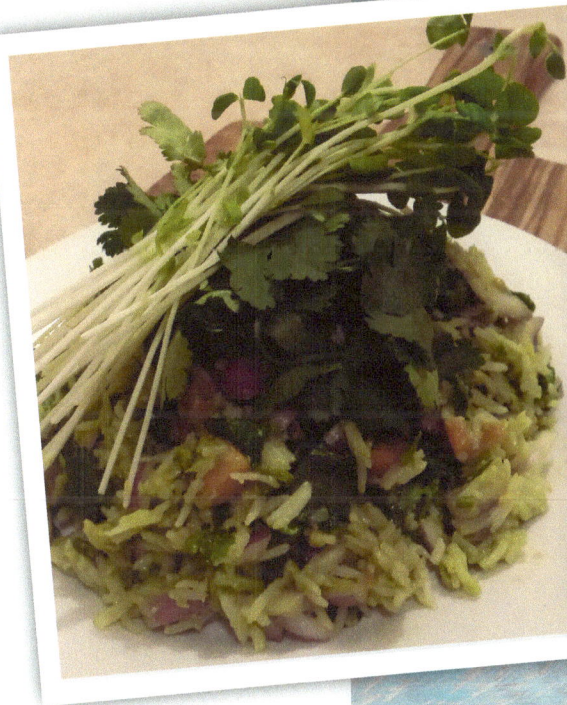

Crispy Tofu and Chilli Stir Fry

Because of my love for hot spices and their incredible health benefits, chilli is right up there on my list! I use chilli in my recipes for many reasons, mostly for flavour, however I came to discover that it does assist in losing that unwanted body fat. I never throw a chilli out – when they start to look like they're losing their freshness, I dry them, seeds and all. They are perfect for making your own chilli powder. Even crushing up the dried chilli to re-plant will grow fresh new chilli in no time.

4 handfuls of fresh baby spinach
4 fresh chillies, finely chopped
1 block organic tofu
2 heaped tbsp raw, cold-pressed organic coconut oil (or 4 tbsp if in its liquid state)
1 generous pinch pink Himalayan salt and cracked black pepper

Chop the tofu into small rectangles or squares, then fry in a wok with the coconut oil until slightly crispy on the outside.
Add the finely chopped chilli with pinch of pink Himalayan salt and cracked black pepper, and stir through.
Just as you are ready to serve, gently mix in the baby spinach.
Coconut oil will ignite the flavours of the chilli, pink Himalayan salt and cracked black pepper through the tofu, complementing the delicate freshness added by the baby spinach.
This is a great dish for quick and easy eating on the run, and takes next to no time at all to prepare.
The natural flavours of the few spices is all the sauce this dish needs.
Enjoy!

Shredded cauliflower tastes great as an alternative to tofu, and you can add a handful of raw almonds for that protein hit.
Optional: a squeeze of fresh lemon over this dish also tastes amazing!

African Mediterranean Inspired Veggies

This simple yet delicate combination has been inspired by my love for culture, and the people of West and South Africa.

3 large tomatoes
3 medium zucchini
1 handful raw walnuts
1 fresh lemon, juiced
1 fresh lime, juiced
1 generous drizzle of pure organic olive oil
1 pinch Himalayan salt
1 pinch cracked black pepper

Cut the tomatoes in half from the sides, not the top, and slice the zucchini into halves.
Cook the zucchini in a non-stick sandwich press until crispy and golden, remove and cook the tomatoes in the same way until soft in the middle and beginning to crisp on the outside.
Place the cooked vegetables in a serving bowl and sprinkle over the walnuts, a generous drizzle of olive oil, the fresh lemon and lime juice, and the pink Himalayan salt and cracked black pepper.
Gently mix together and enjoy!

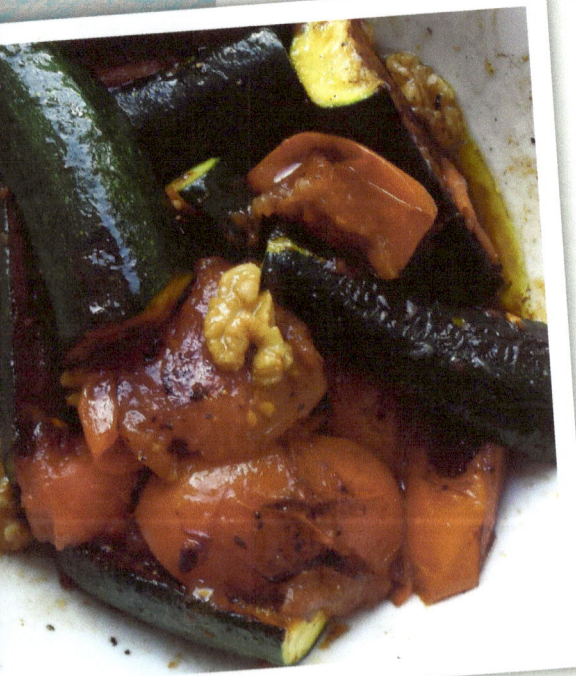

Warm Sweet Potato and Zucchini Medley

This is one of my favourite dishes.

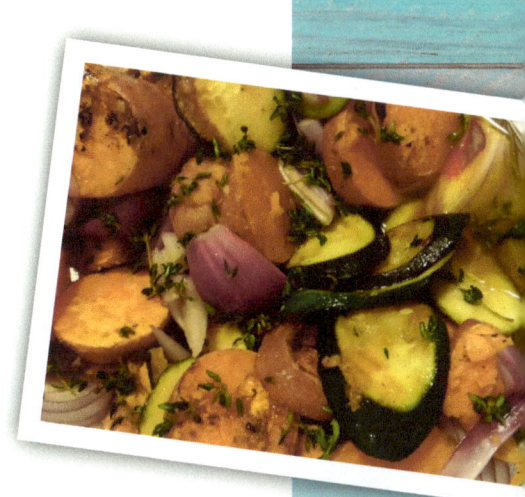

1 large sweet potato
2 large zucchini
1 medium bunch broccoli (optional)
1 purple onion
1 very generous drizzle olive oil
1 generous pinch Himalayan Salt and cracked black pepper
1 handful fresh oregano
1 handful fresh rosemary
1/2 fresh lemon, juiced, or 3 capfuls apple cider vinegar
1 fresh lime, juiced (use pulp as well)

Chop the sweet potato into whatever sized pieces you prefer and cook in a non-stick sandwich press.
Chop zucchini, broccoli and purple onion into pieces, whichever size you like.
When the sweet potato is done, cook the zucchini and broccoli in the sandwich press until slightly golden on the outside.
Place sweet potato, zucchini and broccoli on a serving plate, gently tossing through the purple onion.
Add fresh oregano and rosemary, as well as the juice of the lemon and lime, and the fresh lime pulp.
Gently mix together, along with a generous drizzle of olive oil and sprinkle of pink Himalayan salt and cracked black pepper. Add your choice of protein, or enjoy the sweet flavours on their own. You'll be in healthy heaven.

Indian-Inspired Spice-Infused Lentils (or lean beef) and Fresh Herb Cabbage Cradles

This spice-infused dish was created from my memories of the smells of spice from my childhood. Its fresh herb embrace really tantalizes the senses, creating an eating experience full of happiness. Now that I am living a lifestyle of plant-based eating, I love to enjoy this dish replacing meat with lentils. It sure is an exciting meal to come home to!

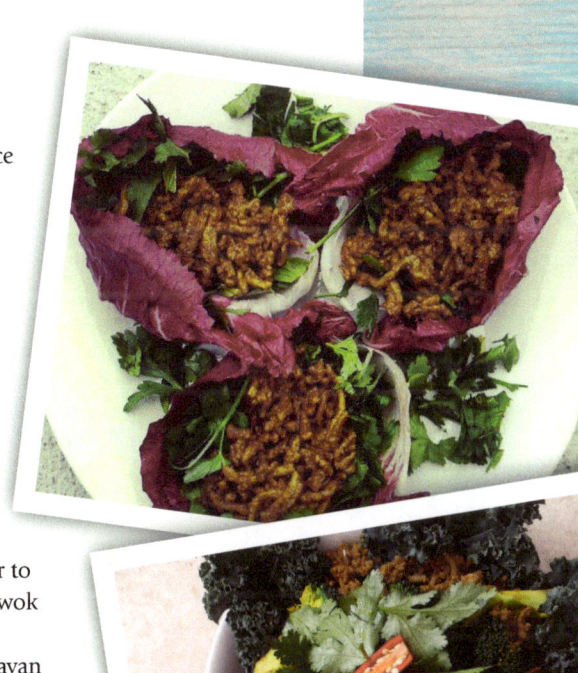

1 purple cabbage
500g lentils (or lean beef that has been minced)
2 heaped tbsp raw, cold-pressed coconut oil (or 4 tbsp if in its liquid state)
1 generous pinch each of organic turmeric powder, cumin powder, paprika, cayenne pepper, pink Himalayan salt and cracked black pepper
1 bunch each of fresh coriander, mint and Italian parsley, finely chopped

Pre-cook the lentils, boiling until almost soft and ready to eat, then transfer to a hot wok and finish off by frying in coconut oil. If using beef, fry in a hot wok with coconut oil.
Add generous pinches of turmeric, cumin, paprika, cayenne pepper, Himalayan salt and cracked black pepper, and mix through well.
Wash as many cabbage leaves as you need and place out on serving tray.
Place the cooked mixture into the cabbage leaves.
Sprinkle the finely chopped coriander, mint and Italian parsley over each cradle, finishing with a squeeze of lemon. Enjoy!
Option: I also use curly kale leaves as an alternative to the purple cabbage. The heat from the cooked lean beef or lentils warms the kale leaf and gives it an amazing taste!

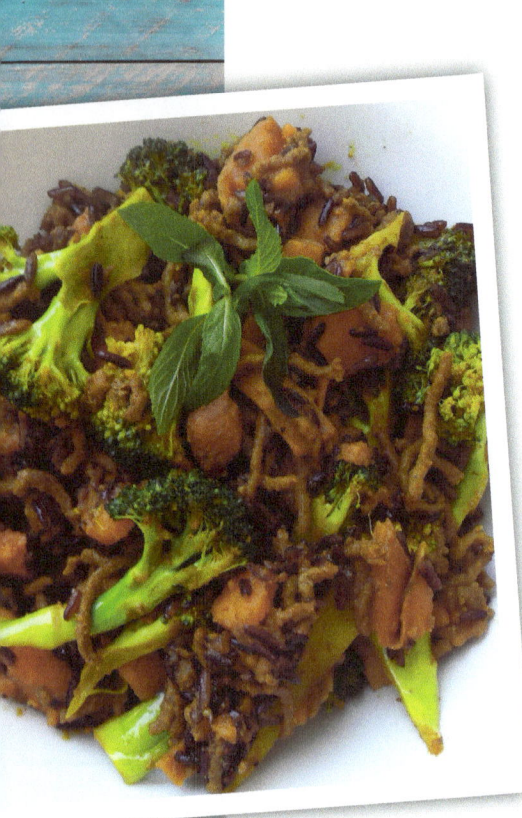

Black Rice, Broccoli, Black Bean (or beef) and Sweet Potato Medley

1 handful fresh mint
1 medium sweet potato
1 small head broccoli
1 cup black rice
1 pinch organic turmeric powder
1 pinch organic cumin powder
2 heaped tbsp raw, cold-pressed coconut oil (4 tbsp if in its liquid state)
400g lean minced beef
Vegetarian option: use lentils or black beans

Cook the rice.
Cook lean beef (or lentils /black beans) in a hot wok with coconut oil.
(If using black beans or lentils you will need to boil them until ready to eat)
Add turmeric and cumin to the wok (add a pinch of cayenne pepper if you're wanting a dash of heat), and mix through well.
While this is cooking, chop the sweet potato and broccoli into small slices.
Place the sweet potato in a non-stick sandwich press to soften, and add the small pieces of broccoli straight into the wok.
When sweet potato is slightly soft, add it to the wok and gently combine.
When rice is completely cooked add it into the wok mixture, also combining gently.
Place on serving dish and garnish with chopped mint.

Wondering why I eat a lot of turmeric and ginger in my meals?

When I eat fresh ginger it fires up my digestive juices and also helps to settle any stomach upset. Fresh ginger is a good friend for relieving joint pain and muscle aches. I absolutely love the stuff! I eat turmeric both fresh and in organic powder form where ever I can in my food because I know how good it is for my whole body, my brain and even my mood. I could go on all day about how amazing turmeric is!

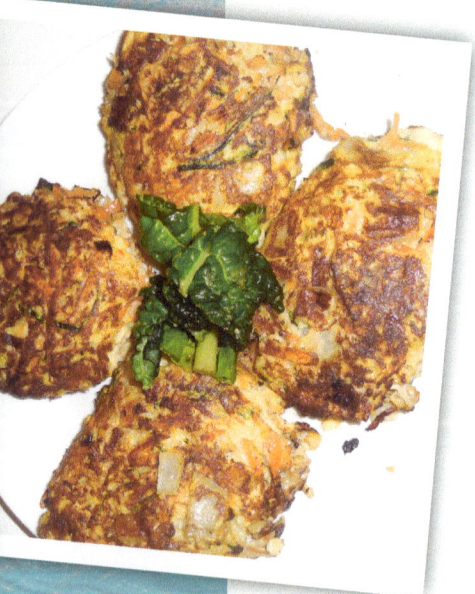

Zucchini Fritters

I'm in love with these zucchini fritters. They are so full of vitality and goodness, and the taste is way too irresistible. I make up a batch of my sweet and spicy chilli sauce (see page 50) to create a delicious flavour hit.

1 large zucchini, grated
1 large sweet potato or yam, grated
1 large onion, diced
2 heaped tbsp raw, cold-pressed coconut oil (4 tbsp in its liquid state)
1 pinch each of pink Himalayan salt and cracked black pepper

Optional extras: fresh corn kernels, tuna chunks in spring water, grated carrot

Mix ingredients together in a bowl with 1 tablespoon of coconut oil.
Shape the mix into patties (along with optional extras if desired). The moistness of the zucchini along with the thickness of the sweet potato helps to act as a glue, keeping the fritters in one piece.
Heat the other tablespoon of coconut oil in a non-stick frying pan and place fritters in, cooking on both sides till golden brown and crisp.
Garnish with pieces of crisp cos lettuce.

Spicy Anaheim Pepper Bruschetta – also known as chiayo chilli or banana chilli

1 large fresh lemon, juiced
1 large carrot, finely diced
1 large purple onion, finely diced
1 large tomato, finely diced
1 bunch fresh coriander, finely diced, stalks included
6 large Anaheim peppers, de-seeded and de-ribbed

Start by making the guacamole (see page 47) then after cutting in half and scooping out the ribs and seeds of the Anaheim peppers, place the guacamole inside the halved peppers. Then add all the other chopped ingredients on top of the guacamole in the Anaheim peppers.

Alternatively – make a batch of smashed avocado (see page 49). Slice peppers in half and lay them onto serving board. Place smashed avocado mixture into each pepper. Sprinkle chopped carrots, chopped purple onion ,chopped tomato and chopped coriander over each pepper. Enjoy!

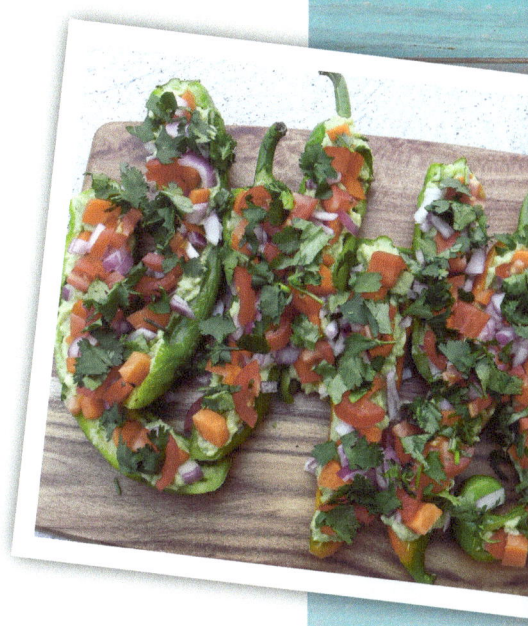

Thai-Inspired Shredded Organic Chicken or Tofu Soup

A great dish to have when a pick me up is needed or if you're not feeling well.
1 organic free-range, pasture-raised chicken breast,
1/2 bunch broccoli , chopped into pieces
1/2 savoy cabbage, shredded
1 bunch fresh coriander, chopped
1 thumb fresh ginger, grated
3 red chilli's, finely chopped
1 fresh lemon, juiced
1 carrot, chopped (optional)
1 pinch pink Himalayan salt
1 pinched cracked black pepper

Vegetarian option: substitute tofu for chicken, but do not boil.

Place the chicken breast in a pot of boiling water and boil for 15-20 minutes. Once done, turn off the heat and put a lid on the pot, leaving the chicken to continue to cook in the residual heat for 45 minutes to an hour. Even when the heat has fully subsided, leave the lid on.
When ready to eat, take out the cooked chicken breast and place on a board. Shred using a fork. Re-heat the juices that are left in the pot.
Take a serving bowl and place in the ginger, chilli, broccoli, and savoy cabbage. Top with the shredded chicken pieces, a sprinkle of pink Himalayan salt and cracked black pepper.
Pour the hot juices from the chicken pot over the ingredients in the serving bowl.
If using tofu as an alternative to chicken, slice the tofu into small blocks and add to ingredients in the serving bowl. Pour over 1 1/2 cups of boiled water and the flavours in the serving bowl will quickly come together forming a soup.
Garnish with fresh coriander and enjoy!

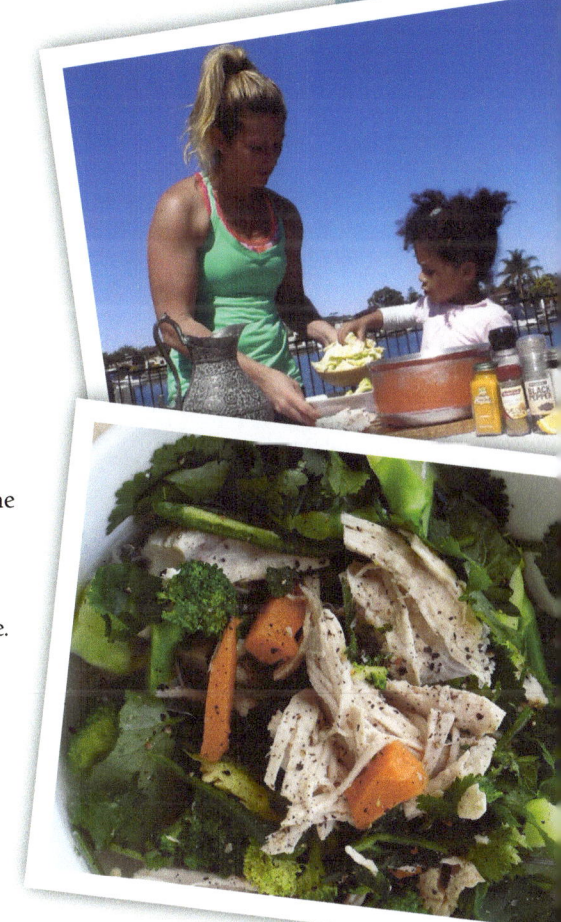

Crunchy Coconut Prawn heads with folded egg, organic cottage or goat cheese and pan fried cherry tomato

I love finding ways to reduce waste and create a meal with food that may have otherwise been discarded. This recipe came about exactly this way and has been inspired by friends of mine and a Chinese-Filipino style meal that they cooked for me. When cooked properly, prawn heads can become crisp and crunchy just like chips and they taste just like prawn crackers! Use this dish when you are planning to eat fresh prawns and try it for yourself

500g fresh prawns
3 free range organic fresh eggs
1 small tub organic cottage cheese
1 small punnet cherry tomatoes
2 heaped tbsp organic-cold pressed coconut oil
1/4 bunch Italian parsley
1 pinch Himalayan salt
1 pinch cracked black pepper

How to cook crispy prawn heads:
Slice horizontally across the prawn head, removing the eyes and the gooey top part of the head.
Remove any excess shell and place the heads in a pre-heated pan that has been drizzled with coconut oil. Face the heads downwards into the pan so that the legs are facing up. Press down on the prawn heads with a turning spatula. This will open the heads up and help them to cook through. Cook on both sides, pressing down with the turning spatula until crispy.

Folding Egg:
Crack three or four free range organic eggs into a bowl and mix together. Turn out mixed eggs onto a small (pancake sized) pre-heated hot non-stick pan drizzled with coconut oil and cook till golden yellow on each side. Use turning spatula to then fold cooked egg in half and lay out on serving plate.

Place the cherry tomatoes into the same pan and cook them until skin slightly softened. Cooking the tomatoes in the same pan will soak up all the delicious flavours, and will only take a few minutes to cook.
Add cooked crispy prawn heads, a large dollop of organic ,GMO free cottage cheese or goats cheese and the cooked cherry tomatoes on to the serving plate.
Sprinkle with Himalayan salt & cracked black pepper. Garnish with fresh Italian parsley. Enjoy!

Keep travelling the road you set out on. It won't always be easy, but it will always be worth it.

Raw Pad Thai with Creamy Cashew Dressing

These flavours spring from memories of the amazing tastes I experienced during my travels in Vietnam.

2 large carrots
1 celeriac, kohlrabi or parsnip
1/2 egg plant
1 large yellow bell pepper
1/4 purple cabbage
1/4 broccoli or 1 large handful fresh green beans
1 lemon or 1 lime
1 thumb size of fresh ginger
1 large handful bean sprouts
1 handful fresh coriander
1 small handful sesame seeds (black or white)
1 pinch paprika
1 pinch Himalayan salt
1 sprinkle crushed peanuts (optional)

Julienne the carrot, parsnip (or kohlrabi or celeriac) eggplant, yellow bell pepper, purple cabbage, and fresh ginger. Slice the broccoli into tiny pieces, or use whole green beans.

Create the creamy cashew dressing (see page 47).
Mix the dressing through all ingredients. Place on a large serving plate. Garnish with sesame seeds, crushed peanuts, bean sprouts and fresh coriander. Enjoy!

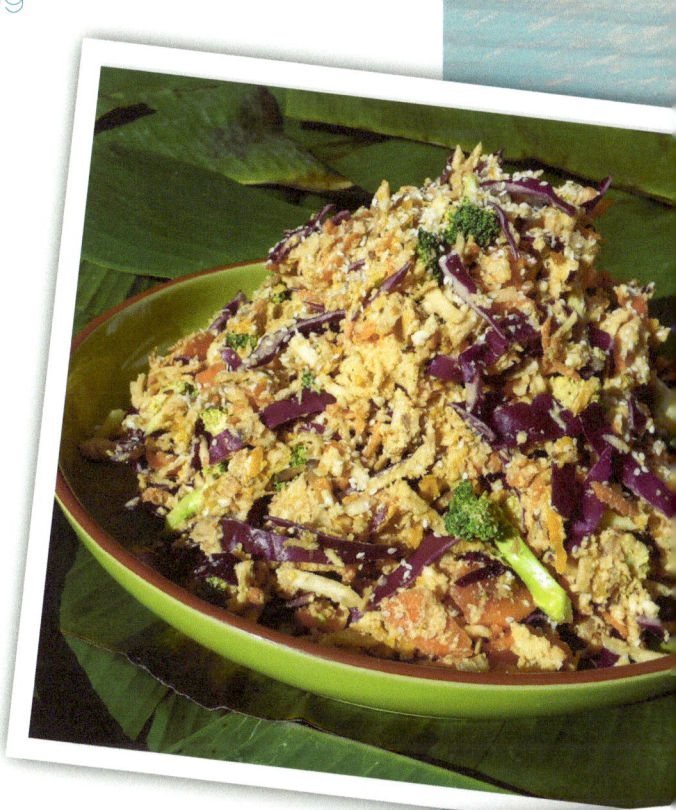

Warm Rainbow Carrot Medley

1 bunch organic rainbow carrots (around 8–10), top stems removed
1/2 head broccoli, cut into pieces
1 handful fresh mint leaves, chopped
1 handful fresh rosemary, chopped
1 handful fresh thyme, chopped
1 pinch cracked black pepper
1 pinch of pink Himalayan salt and cracked black pepper
2 capfuls raw apple cider vinegar
1 drizzle organic olive oil

Place whole carrots into a non-stick sandwich press and cook until soft on the inside and golden on the outside (carrots taste beautiful when pressed and cooked this way).
Place broccoli pieces into the sandwich press and cook lightly.
In a serving dish, add warm cooked carrots and broccoli pieces. Sprinkle over freshly chopped mint, rosemary and thyme along with a pinch of Himalayan salt and cracked black pepper. Add the raw apple cider vinegar and olive oil and combine all ingredients together. Enjoy! This carrot medley goes well with goat cheese and quinoa.

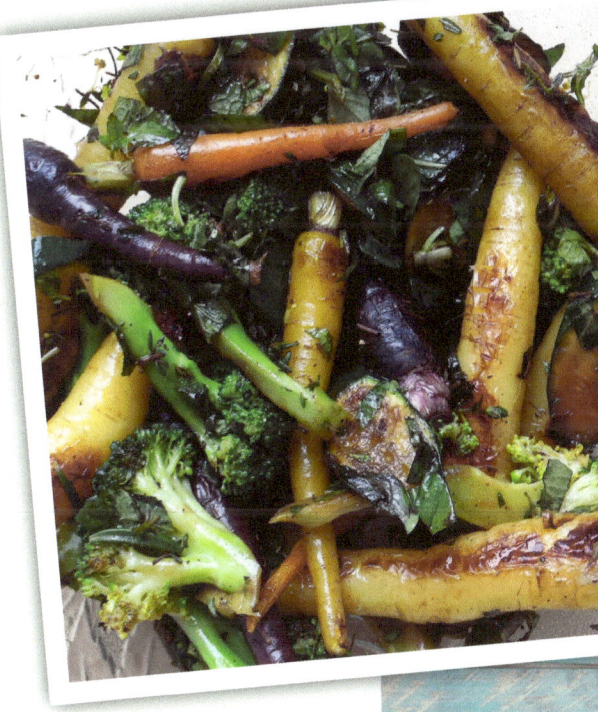

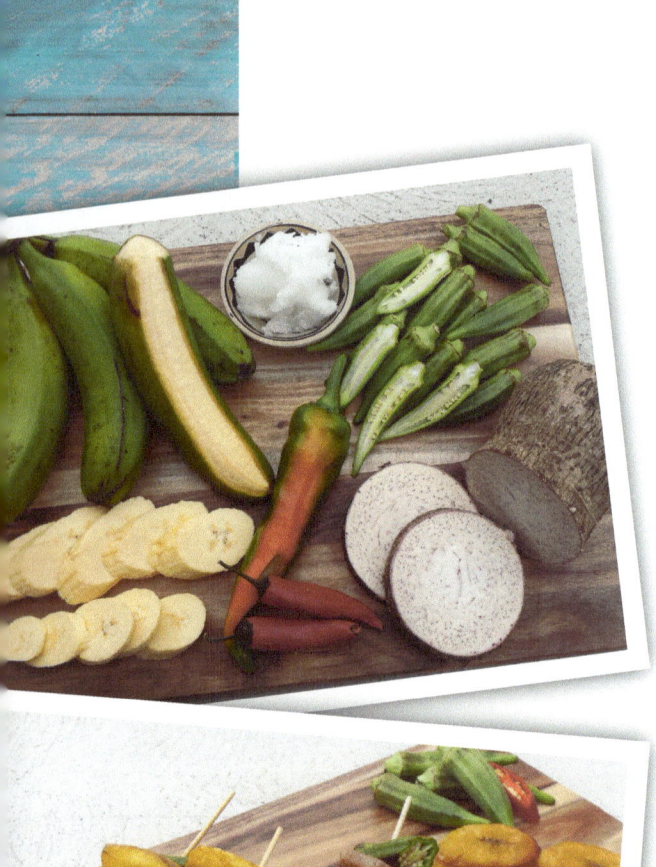

Plantain Skewers with Okra, Poached Crisped Yam, Red Peppers, Raw Honey and Himalayan salt

These tastes of West Africa take me back every time I indulge in these divine flavours. My plantain skewers can easily be eaten as a snack or turned into a main meal, just add a bowl of hearty brown rice or legumes

*Did you know that plantain, and parts of the plantain plant, can be used as a natural fighter against itches and dermatitis? I saw this at work first-hand during my time spent with the locals in the beautiful Islands of Fiji, as well as my time in Africa.

1 yam
2 plantain
300g okra (around 12-15 fresh okra)
3 red chilli
2 tbsp raw honey
3 heaped tbsp raw-cold pressed coconut oil (or 6 if in its liquid form)
2 pinches Himalayan salt
1 packet bamboo skewer sticks

YAM - Cut the yam into large slices, remove the outer skin, then wash the slices. Cut the yam slices into quarters. Place in saucepan and cover with water. Boil for around 20 minutes on a medium heat or until you can easily push a fork through the pieces. Drain the yam well and place in an oven dish that has been pre-coated with coconut oil. Cook in a preheated oven at 180 for five to ten minutes until crisp, turning occasionally. Alternatively, place the yam pieces in a non stick sandwich press to crisp for five minutes, also turning occasionally.

PLANTAIN - Slit plantains with a knife and remove the skin, then chop into pieces. Lay out on a lined tray if cooking in the oven. Drizzle coconut oil over all plantain pieces. Cook in pre-heated oven at 180 degrees for 20 minutes or until golden and crispy. Keep a close eye on the plantain and turn pieces over occasionally to ensure crispy cooking on both sides. If cooking plantain in a sandwich press, brush with coconut oil and turn regularly until crispy on both sides.

OKRA - Rinse okra and slice each one in half. Place sliced okra onto sandwich press and brush with coconut oil. Cook for around five minutes or until slightly crisp, turning occasionally. If cooking in the oven, place on lined tray and cook in a pre-heated oven at 180 degrees for five minutes, turning occasionally until slightly crispy.

RED CHILLI - Slice into small pieces.

Thread the yam, plantain and okra pieces, along with the red chilli slices onto skewer sticks. Sprinkle with Himalayan salt and drizzle with raw honey.

Pizza of Health

You can add all sorts of toppings to your pizza, this is how I do mine.

BASE:
1/2 cauliflower, grated
1 cup psyllium husk
1 generous sprinkle of pink Himalayan salt
1/2 cup sesame seeds, lightly roasted (I roast them in a pre-heated oven at 180 degress for six to seven minutes)
1 cup pepitas, also lightly roasted
1 1/4 cups purified water
Melt 1 to 1 1/2 cups of raw cold pressed coconut oil

Mix together base ingredients and spread over a non-stick pizza tray, pressing and molding it firmly into the tray. Cook the pizza base at 180 degrees in a pre-heated oven for 15 minutes, or until golden and crispy.

Toppings: goat cheese, Kalamata pitted olives, green and orange bell peppers or capsicum, fresh basil, fresh coriander, red habanero chilli peppers. You can also use smashed avocado (see page 49) as a sauce or spread on top of the pizza base before adding the toppings.

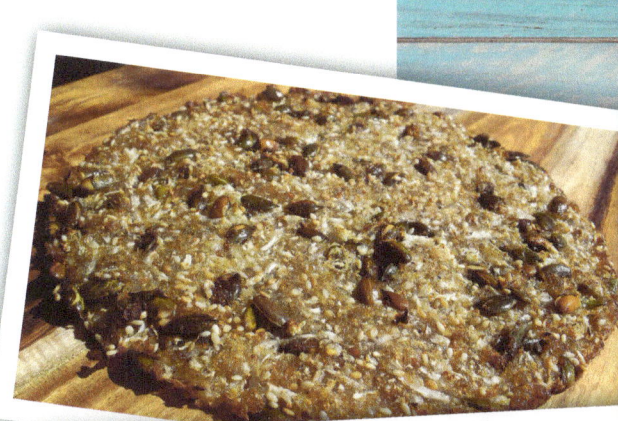
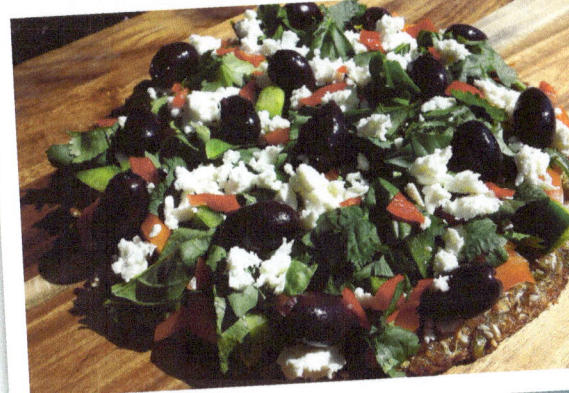

Spicy Tuna Bolognese

My tuna Bolognese can be eaten with quinoa, lentils or brown rice. For spaghetti tuna Bolognese, I like to use a spiralised zucchini or cucumber and mix that through as my spaghetti alternative – it's delicious.

400g fresh tuna pieces, or tuna in spring water
1 onion, peeled and diced
2 jalapenos, thinly sliced with stalks removed
2 cloves of garlic, peeled and thinly diced
3 ripe tomatoes, finely diced
1/2 ripe avocado for cooling option, or sliced cucumber pieces
1 sprinkle of pink Himalayan salt
1 sprinkle of cracked black pepper
1 tbsp raw, cold-pressed organic coconut oil

Preheat a non-stick frying pan with coconut oil.
Add onion, garlic and jalapenos, then add tomatoes and continue to stir.
Place tuna pieces into the mixture and gently combine the flavours together until cooked. Sprinkle Himalayan salt and cracked black pepper into the cooked mixture and stir.
Place on a serving dish with avocado or cucumber pieces on the side and enjoy this delicious meal!

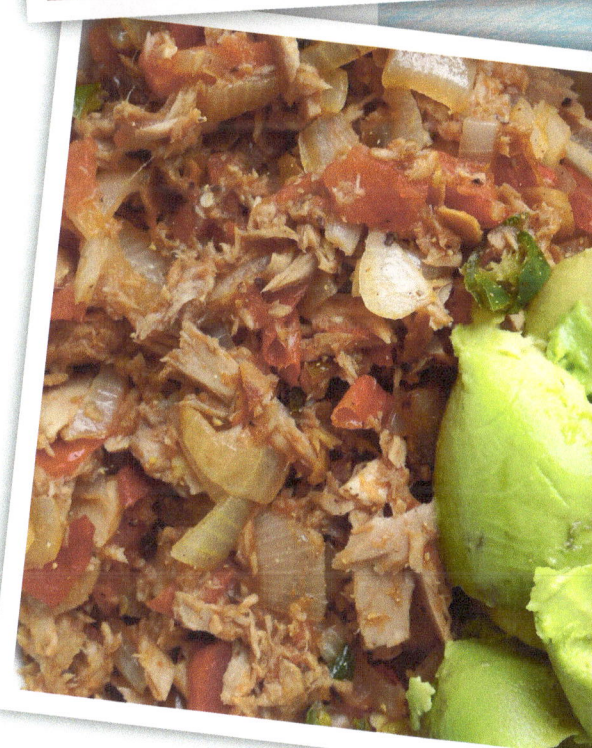

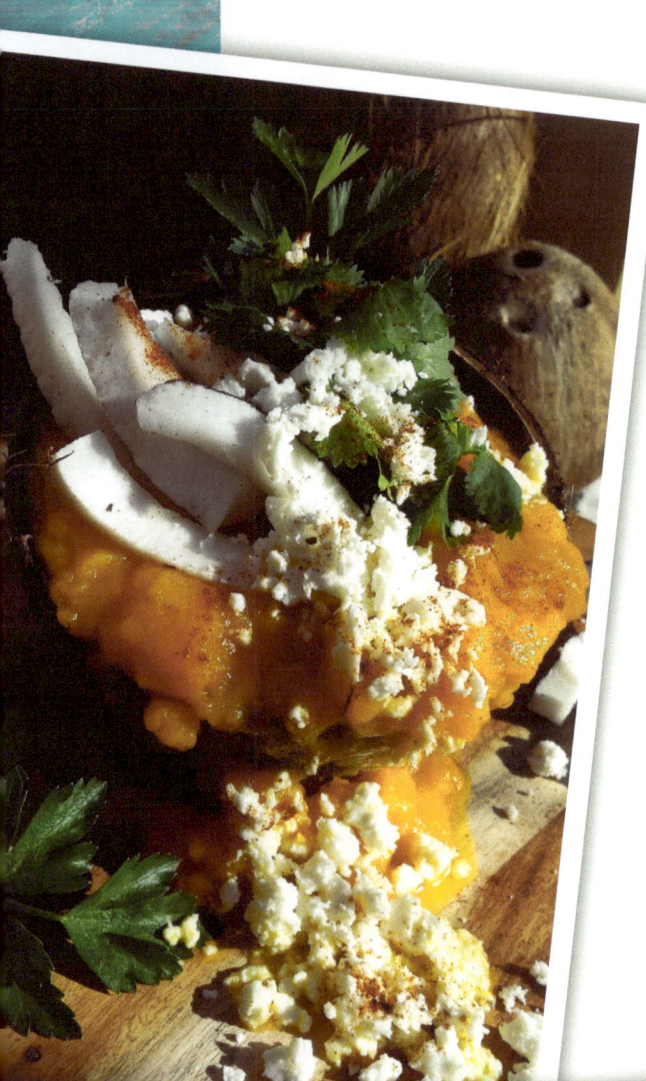

Coconut Pumpkin Soup

This delicious and easy to make coconut pumpkin soup was inspired by my time in the islands of Fiji. I hope you enjoy this as much as I do.

1 pumpkin of choice, skin washed and kept on, chopped into chunks and boiled in pot of hot water till soft
Place the cooked pumpkin in a blender and blend till smooth adding:
1 cup pure organic coconut cream
1 tiny sprinkle of nutmeg
1 sprinkle turmeric powder
1 sprinkle of paprika
1 sprinkle of cayenne pepper (optional if wanting a bit of heat!)
1 sprinkle Himalayan salt
1 sprinkle cracked black pepper

Blend ingredients together well.
Serve with a garnish of fresh coconut flesh, fresh parsley and a sprinkle of goats cheese – enjoy!

Note: this pumpkin soup recipe can be used as a base for a stew-like dish. I add chunky baked veggies and crispy tofu pieces into the pumpkin soup and it tastes delicious. I also use this pumpkin soup recipe to cook lentils with too, again adding my choice of veggies. You can even use this recipe in a healthy wholesome wholemeal risotto. If you prefer animal proteins you can add lean meat or chicken pieces with lots of fresh herbs when using this recipe in a stew.

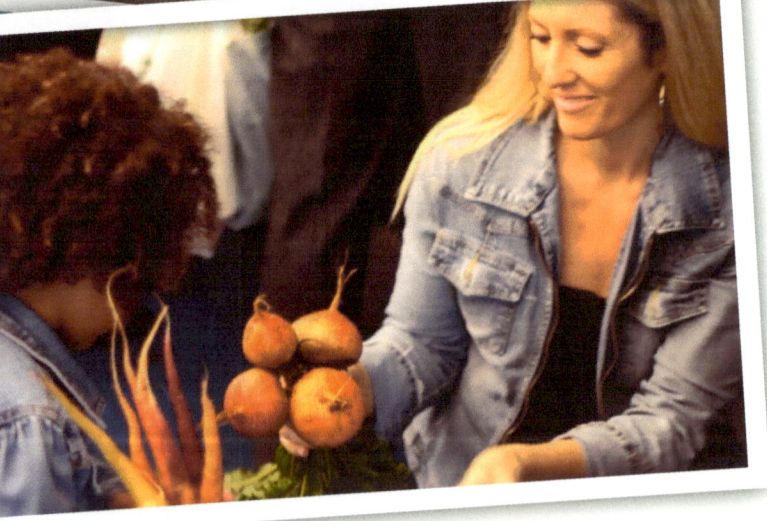

Sometimes life will try to turn your world upside down. Look for a way to fight back. There is always a way around. Never give up!

Adore Salads

Get to know your local farmers and growers. Finding out where your food comes from, and how it is grown, is really important. I make sure my organic produce falls under the strict certified organic standards, because a lot of food companies use the words 'organic' and 'natural' when actually it's not. It always pays to do a bit of research for the sake of your health. I started by searching out local growers markets and community gardens, and even local produce swaps with local harvest. You can learn so much from talking to the growers, and you never know what you might discover. The organic fresh produce that arrives in your hand not long after it has been picked makes all the difference in quality, fresh eating, not to mention health and wellness. Better still, try growing your own fresh produce at home, it's so rewarding and therapeutic.

Nutritious salads are a great way to fill up. I eat a huge bowl of salad daily – it's one way I cleanse my system, alongside other methods such as green juice and lots of water. I just can't get enough of dark leafy greens, the more the better. There are so many ways to create delicious tasting salads and make sure dark leafy greens are finding their way into your system. I always make my own dressings. That way I know exactly what I'm eating and can be sure I'm receiving all the benefits of the nutrients, vitamins and minerals dark leafy greens hold. There is no point eating a beautiful salad if you are going to smother it with sugar filled dressings that are often lathered with chemical ingredients, defeating the point of the dark leafy greens you're about to eat. I take pride in nourishing myself, and I encourage you to do the same. I've created some delicious ways to keep exciting tastes and goodness alive in my salads, along with natural healthy dressings. Keep in mind that all these salads work well as a meal on their own, or accompanying a main dish.

You can get creative with my salad recipes, experiment with them and even try to create your own versions. With salad the sky really is the limit.

Avocado and Beetroot Salad with Eggplant Crisps

This salad recipe came about one day when my daughter wanted to eat fresh raw beetroot just like you would an apple. We often include fresh beetroot in our weekly supply that we get from our local organic farmers and growers. I decided to create a salad that highlights the sweet flavours of fresh beetroot. Fresh raw beetroot is so good for liver cleansing, and I use it in a lot of my juices too (see page 16).

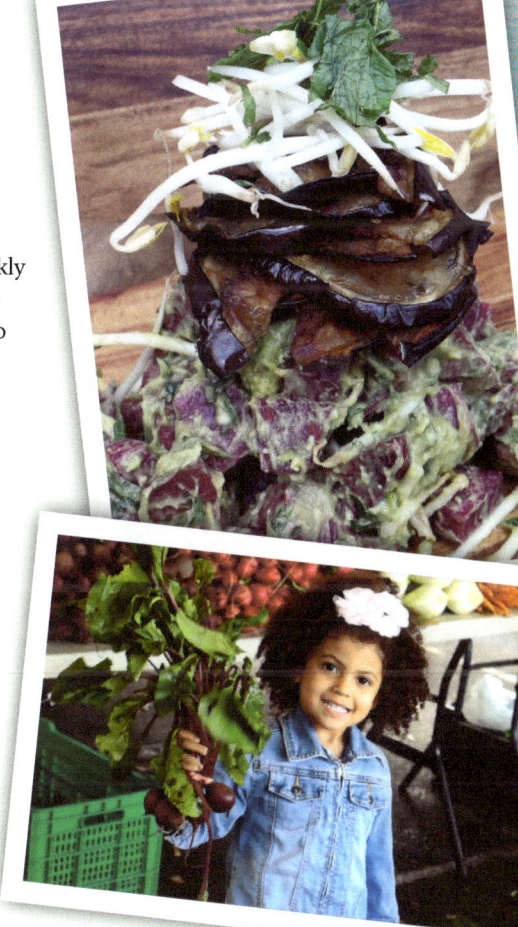

You will need:
1 eggplant (see page 61) on how to prepare eggplant crisps
2 fresh beetroot, washed and diced, skin kept on
1 handful fresh bean sprouts
2 handfuls fresh mint, finely chopped , keep 1 handful aside to use for garnish
1 avocado, seed removed

Scoop avocado into a blender or mini chopper, adding 1 handful of the fresh mint with a pinch of Himalayan salt and a generous drizzle of olive oil. Blend together. You can also add a squeeze of fresh lemon or lime here into the blended avocado mix if desired.
Place diced beetroot into a bowl and add the avocado mix, combining and stirring it thoroughly, then place onto a serving board.
Place eggplant crisps on top of the beetroot salad, and garnish with fresh bean sprouts and the remaining fresh mint. Enjoy!
Optional: this also tastes great with my garlic sauce (see page 48) as an alternative to the avocado dressing.

Deconstructed Bruschetta Yellow Bell Pepper Boats

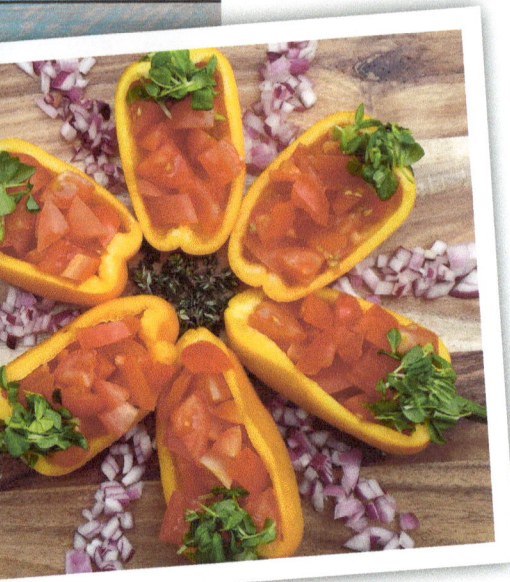

Bruschetta is an all time favourite of mine, but eating it with a healthy, nourishing option as the base, rather than a heavy bread, is even better. This is such a fun way to enjoy eating bruschetta, and to get creative with super healthy herbs and vegetables. I often eat this salad of an evening with a sprinkle of crushed raw almonds or pepitas for extra crunch and a hit of protein. I like to arrange my deconstructed bruschetta yellow bell pepper boats in a decorative display to add even more interest and excitement to this salad.

3 yellow bell peppers (also commonly known as capsicum)
2 large tomatoes
1 purple onion
1/2 bunch freshly chopped coriander
1/4 bunch finely chopped fresh oregano
1 pinch pink Himalayan salt
1 pinch cracked black pepper
1 sprinkle cumin
1 lime, cut in half
1 generous drizzle olive oil

Cut yellow bell peppers in half and remove the seeds and ribs.
Arrange the cut yellow bell pepper halves in a circle on a serving board.
Finely chop the tomato and place inside the pepper halves.
Finely dice purple onion and arrange in between the peppers.
Place chopped fresh coriander at top ends of the yellow bell peppers
Place fresh oregano in the centre.
Sprinkle pink Himalayan salt, black cracked pepper and cumin over the top for taste.
Optional: you can add finely chopped serrano chillies or jalapeno (stems, ribs, seeds removed) for less or more spice to taste, and crushed almonds or pepitas for crunch.
Squeeze over the juice of the lime and drizzle over a generous amount of olive oil.
I also love to eat this dish with my home made guacamole (see page 47) or tahini (see page 48) splashed over the top. Enjoy!

Golden Beet, Fresh Basil and Cashew Salad

This really is such a delicious sweet-tasting salad. The golden beets make this dish so flavoursome, the hint of basil splashed throughout and that crunch of cashew adding a special something to the whole experience.

4 golden beetroot, grated
1 large parsnip, grated
2 large handfuls of fresh basil, roughly chopped
1 bunch coriander, finely chopped
1 generous handful raw cashews

Mix all together then add dressing of your choice, I like to add the following dressing combination to this particular salad.
1 tbsp tahini, 1/2 cup olive oil, generous pinch of Himalayan salt and cracked black pepper, juice of 1 fresh lemon and its pulp. Combine all ingredients and then drizzle over the salad. It leaves you feeling light, satisfied and energized after eating.
Optional: this salad is great with organic black rice mixed through to make it warmer. It gives that real rustic authentic flavour, highlighted by the golden beets and fresh herbs!

Warm Kumara and Golden Beet Salad

Colour makes food so inviting and to me this is what makes this salad so appealing. If you're struggling with eating good nourishing food, a fantastic way to solve this is to make healthy look great! This salad sure does that! I serve this on a large board so the vibrant colours can be laid out and fully appreciated. This salad just makes eating for health all the more enjoyable. Of course you can add your own textures and tastes to this salad as you desire - crushed walnuts, scrambled tofu, organic chicken pieces from appropriate sources, even avocado -but for me this is the way I most enjoy my warm kumara and golden beet salad.

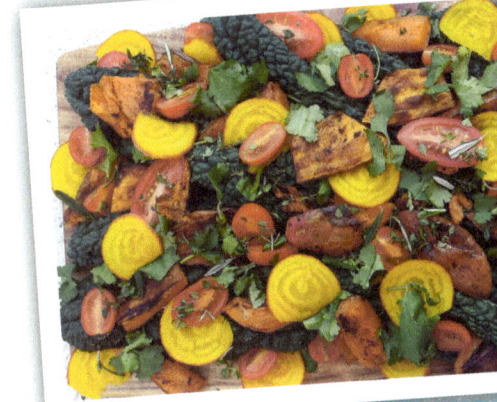

1 large kumara cut into thick pieces and cooked in a non stick sandwich press until crispy on the outside
1 bunch Tuscan kale, washed and laid out on serving board
1 punnet grape tomatoes, cut into halves
1 large golden beetroot, thinly sliced
1 handful fresh chopped coriander
1 small handful fresh rosemary leaves
1 small handful freshly chopped thyme
1 lime, freshly squeezed

Spread all ingredients over the Tuscan kale leaves and drizzle fresh lime juice over the salad. Finish with a large drizzle of olive oil and a pinch of Himalayan salt and cracked black pepper. Enjoy!

Purple Cabbage Salad Bowls and Wraps

These taste great and are easy to whip up for a quick, enticing meal. You can add whatever you want for the filling, the more colour the better. Be creative with the fresh ingredients you already have. I regularly keep fresh produce in my kitchen and I use what fresh produce I have on hand at the time to create the filling. It's amazing what you can come up with! This is a delicious, light and satisfying meal. Here is what I used to create my nourishing filling...

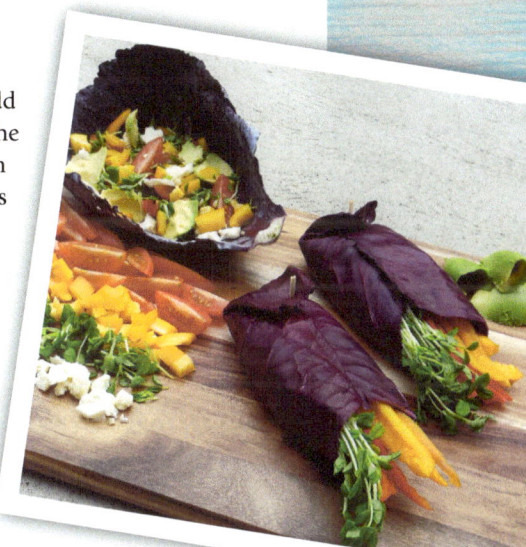

1 fresh purple cabbage - use 1 whole cabbage leaf per salad bowl or wrap
1 red capsicum
1 yellow capsicum or fresh corn kernels
1/4 cauliflower
1 bunch snow pea sprouts
1 ripe avocado
1 punnet grape or cherry tomatoes
1 bunch coriander, or fresh herbs of your choice

Salad Bowl: chop tomatoes, cauliflower, red capsicum, yellow capsicum (or use fresh corn kernel pieces), snow pea sprouts, coriander (or fresh herbs of your choice) into small pieces and place in cabbage leaves. I like to have avocado two ways in these salad bowls and wraps.
One way is to simply cut the avocado in half, remove the seed, scoop out the flesh with a small spoon and place small scoops of the avocado in the cabbage leaf. Alternatively, you can spread the ripe avocado over the cabbage leaf first to act as a spread before adding all the other ingredients. My smashed avocado (see page 49) also works nicely with these.
Wraps: place all chopped ingredients inside cabbage leaf, fold both sides in and then fold up one end and secure with a toothpick. Drizzle sauce of choice over the top for extra satisfaction.
If wanting animal proteins, 250g of tuna in spring water, a boiled organic, free-range and pasture-raised egg cut into slices, or even 250g grilled chicken pieces.

Green Sprout and Lime Salad

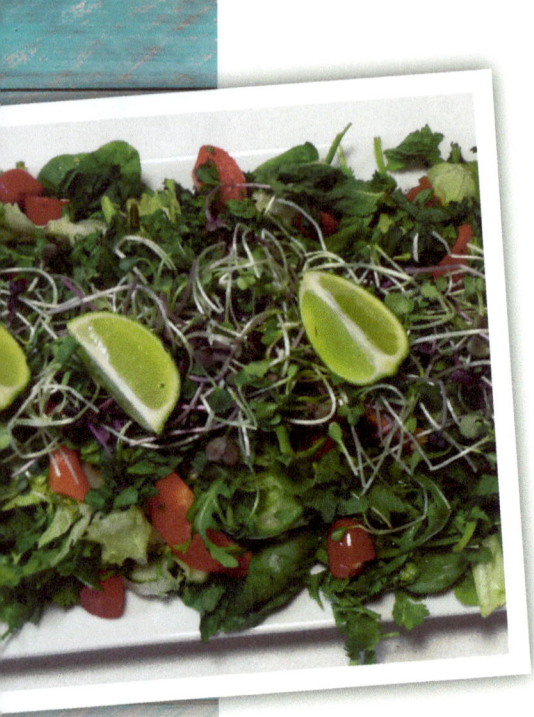

I often create my salads purely from the fresh ingredients in my fridge at the time, and it's great to know that my weekly fresh green stock up is being put to its maximum use, giving me all its benefits and never wasted. Even If some of my greens are looking a little tired, or just not ticking the fresh box for my salad, I juice them. Either way I make sure those greens are getting into my system one way or another. Greens are such an important daily necessity, especially for maintaining overall health in the long run.

For my green sprout and lime salad I use:
1 red capsicum, cut into slices
1 fresh lime, cut into wedges
1 handful fresh watercress
1/2 cos lettuce, chopped
2 large handfuls baby spinach
1 bunch fresh coriander, finely chopped
1/2 bunch fresh mint, finely chopped
1/2 bunch cilantro or Italian parsley, finely chopped
1 large handful fresh rocket
2 large handfuls sunflower sprouts

Combine all the ingredients by laying them out on a serving plate, and drizzle over one of my favourite dressing recipes or simply just a good splash of olive oil, balsamic vinegar and a squeeze of fresh lime juice, with a sprinkle of pink Himalayan salt or cracked black pepper – it's so delicious and refreshing!

Healing Herb and Mixed Kale Salad

I love to combine the flavours of numerous herbs and explore the six tastes. In just one mouthful the six tastes of sweet, sour, salty, bitter, pungent, and astringent sensations can be experienced, all exploding in your mouth at the same time! I really treasure the importance of taste in my food. It's incredible how our taste buds unlock the nutritive value of foods, and provide the initial spark to the entire digestive process. I use herbs because it's one of the best ways to create many exciting natural tastes and flavours in my food.

Another unique quality of herbs is the amazing health and healing properties they provide. I try to eat a variety of fresh herbs daily for that reason alone. My herb salad was created for the purpose of extinguishing a deep re-occurring cough that my daughter was suffering from. I use fresh rosemary to help relieve coughs. Sage is an ideal herb for sore throats.

Using several types of fresh herbs together or even using herbs and spices together actually has even more benefits. I often use rosemary in combination with thyme and sage for increased health benefits and added flavour. My daughter actually asks me for fresh rosemary leaves to chew on and eat while we make this salad together! It's a wonderful salad for taste, health and healing.

Combine 1 large handful each of:
Fresh rocket, oregano, sage, basil, coriander, rosemary, thyme, mint, red Russian kale and Siberian kale.
Drizzle over a generous amount of organic olive oil or flax seed oil, 2 to 3 capfuls of apple cider vinegar, and a sprinkle of Himalayan salt and cracked black pepper.
Optional: add a squeeze of fresh lemon or lime juice, or a small drizzle of organic balsamic vinegar.

This salad is fabulous to have on its own, but also works well accompanying many a savoury dish. Occasionally I like to sprinkle raw almonds, pepitas, macadamias or fresh pomegranate into this salad.

Spiralized Carrot Grilled Chicken and Sesame Salad

This recipe was inspired by my daughter's love for crunchy carrots and fresh basil. Tofu is a great alternative to use in this salad in place of chicken.

1 large carrot, spiralized
1 organic chicken breast, or block tofu grilled (or cooked in non stick sandwich press as I like to do) and cut into pieces
1/2 cup sesame seeds, slightly roasted in a 200 degrees pre-heated oven for 5 min or till slightly golden
1 large handful fresh basil, chopped
1 ripe avocado, seed removed and avocado scooped out with a teaspoon
1 red capsicum, chopped with stem and seeds removed
1 generous drizzle olive oil
1 pinch pink Himalayan salt
1 pinch cracked black pepper

Place spiralized carrot into a salad bowl adding red capsicum, fresh basil and sesame seeds and combine.
Add cooked chicken or tofu pieces, drizzle over olive oil with pinch of Himalayan salt and cracked black pepper to taste, then gently incorporate some scoops of avocado and enjoy!
Optional: fresh grilled fish also works well with this salad!

Zucchini Tahini Salad

This is one of my all time favourite salads. I often make up a big batch of this to last me two or three days. It's so much easier to dive into a healthy meal option if it's there at hand, rather than falling for the temptation of eating junk.

1 sweet potato, chopped into medium sized pieces, grill, oven roast or cook in non stick sandwich press till soft
1 handful raw walnuts
1/2 punnet cherry tomatoes, cut into halves
1/2 bunch fresh Chinese watercress, chopped
1 zucchini spiralized
1 generous drizzle olive oil
2 large tbsp tahini
1 pinch Himalayan salt
1 pinch cracked black pepper

Combine spiralized zucchini, walnuts, cherry tomatoes, tahini, olive oil, Himalayan salt and cracked black pepper into a salad bowl and mix together.
Gently fold through the cooked sweet potato pieces and Chinese watercress.
Optional: I like to add a squeeze of fresh lemon juice!

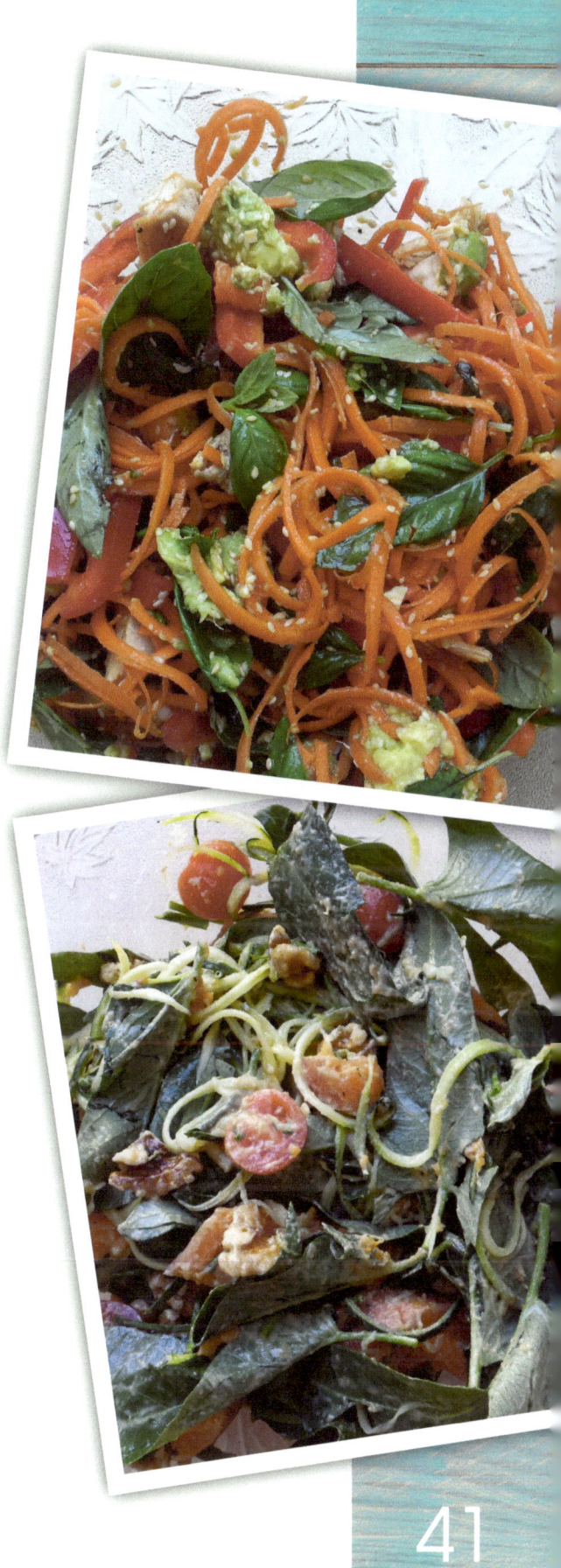

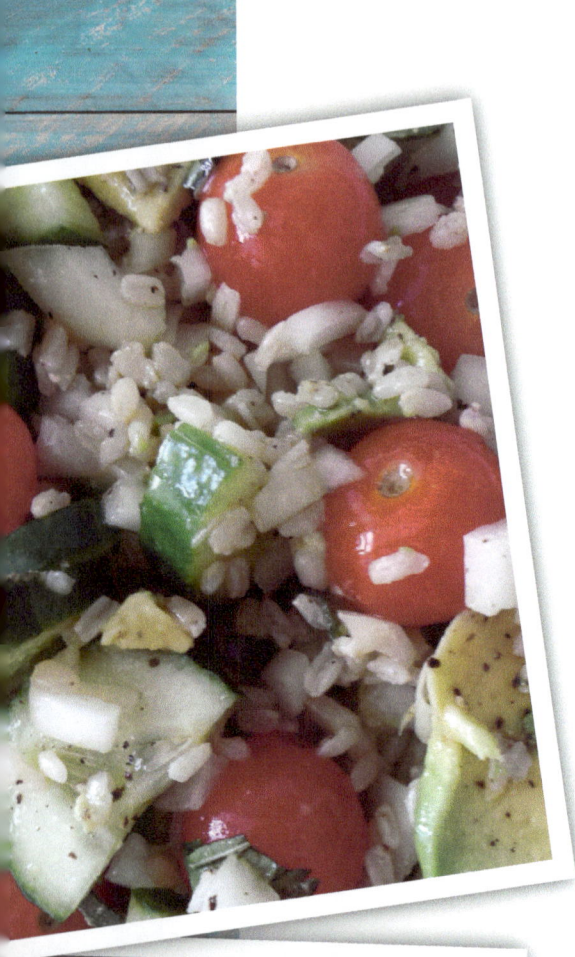

Egyptian Inspired Barley, Fennel and Cucumber Salad

I was privileged to visit Egypt as a young child. I recall the roadside stops for food in desert areas, and the delicious smells and flavours being prepared. This was one very clear starting point for me, where my love of culture, cooking and healthy nourishing food was ignited. The spices and grains I watched the Egyptians cook with captivated me. This salad is a tiny piece of those memories brought to life, but with a splash of Australian influence!

1 cup hulled barley, cooked
1 Lebanese cucumber, diced
1 punnet cherry tomatoes
1 ripe avocado, seed removed and sliced into small pieces
1 onion, finely diced
1/4 fresh fennel bulb, finely chopped
1 bunch fresh dill, finely chopped
1 large drizzle olive oil
1 pinch pink Himalayan salt and cracked black pepper
Optional: add any other fresh finely chopped herbs of your choice

Cook the barley in water in a hot saucepan. Bring to the boil, then simmer on the heat. Place a lid on the saucepan and continue to cook barley till done – approximately 40 minutes. The barley will be done when it has tripled in volume and is soft and chewy. You may need to add more water as the barley will over cook and stick if the pan becomes dry. Check every five minutes until cooked to desired softness. Drain when cooked. Combine cooked barley, finely chopped fennel, fresh dill, cherry tomatoes, onion, Himalayan salt and cracked black pepper (and any other optional fresh herbs) into a serving bowl.
Add drizzle of olive oil and mix through, then gently fold through pieces of avocado and enjoy!

Easy Summer Cooler Salad

This basic salad is sometimes all you need to get the goodness of dark leafy greens and fresh veggies into you. All you need for this salad is:

1 large carrot, chopped into medium-sized pieces
1 cucumber, chopped (I like to use the Lebanese cucumber for its sweeter flavour)
1/2 bunch lacinato kale (or dinosaur kale), chopped into medium-sized pieces
1 large celery stalk, chopped into medium-sized pieces
Combine all ingredients together in a salad bowl. Enjoy!

I like to whip up some of my lemon citrus vinaigrette (see page 49) to pour over this easy salad.
This salad doesn't have to be fancy, although you can easily dress this salad up with some amazing fresh herbs, goat's cheese, olives , fresh beetroot and even fresh corn kernels if so desired.

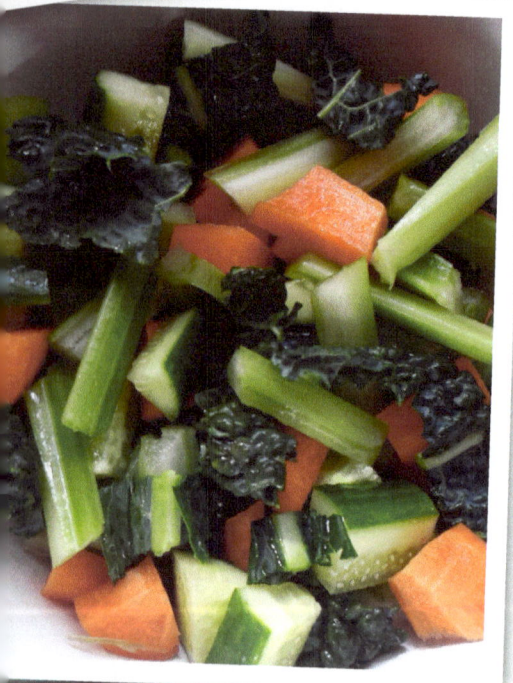

Warm Chickpea Rainbow Salad

For this salad I soak 2 cups of chickpeas in water overnight, then boil them in a saucepan until soft, which usually takes me 30 – 45 minutes on high heat.

While the chickpeas are cooking, I prepare:
1 each of red, yellow and green capsicums, chopped into small pieces and mixed together in a bowl with a drizzle of olive oil, a squeeze of fresh lime, and a pinch of Himalayan salt and cracked black pepper
1 bunch fresh mint, finely chopped
1 bunch English spinach

Lay out the English spinach leaves on serving plate.
Add freshly chopped mint into the chopped up capsicums and place the mixture on top of the laid out spinach leaves
When the chickpeas are cooked, drain them and place in a bowl, together with the chickpeas on top of the capsicum and garnish with oil and fresh mint. I whip up a batch of my fresh tomato and bay leaf sauce (see page 51) and pour this all over. Enjoy!

Tabouleh Avocado Boats

This is a perfect way to get the heart-healthy compounds and nutrients of avocado into your system.

1 ripe avocado cut in half vertically, seed removed (scoop a tiny bit of extra avocado out from each boat to allow a deeper bowl for the tabouleh filling to sit in)

Tabouleh filling :
1/2 cup raw walnuts, crushed
1 handful fresh Italian parsley, finely diced
1 tomato, finely diced
1 purple onion, finely diced
Optional: 1 handful fresh mint, finely diced

In a bowl, mix tabouleh filling together with a drizzle of olive oil, a squeeze of fresh lemon and a pinch of Himalayan salt
Scoop tabouleh mixture into avocado boats, serve and enjoy!
The unique texture that the crushed walnuts provide is delicious!
Couscous can also be used if a more traditional style tabouleh is desired.

Avocado and Sweet Basil Salad

So simple yet so yummy!

1 ripe avocado
1 bunch fresh basil
1 punnet cherry tomatoes

Dress with my lemon citrus vinaigrette (see page 49), or a simple drizzle of olive oil, a tiny splash of balsamic vinegar and a pinch of pink Himalayan salt and cracked black pepper adds the finishing touches. Fold all ingredients together on a serving plate and enjoy!

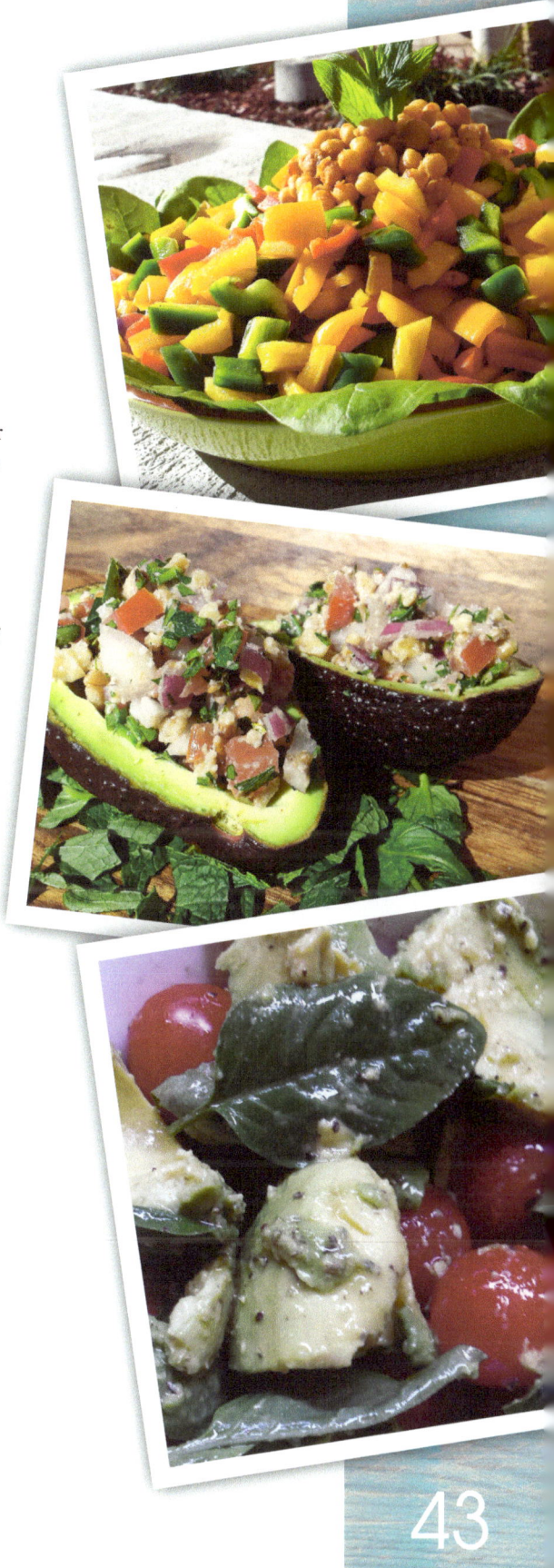

Persist daily – it will bring results even if you don't notice them straight away

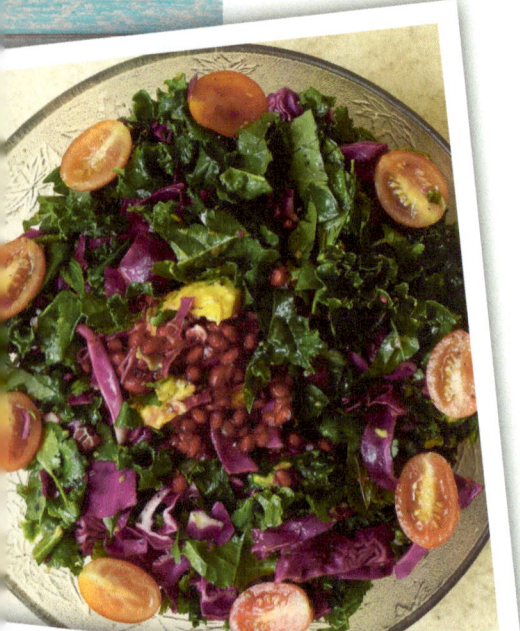

Pomegranate, Purple Cabbage and Fresh crispy Kale Salad

It has been said that kale is like a best friend in the world of greens, especially dark leafy greens, which are some of the most nutrient-dense foods around, providing fibre, minerals, vitamins and antioxidants. This salad is bursting with dark leafy green goodness, vibrant colour and loads of natural flavours. An easy salad to quickly put together with loads of flavour and crunch.

Seeds of 1 pomegranate
1 bunch dark green leafy kale, chopped
1 avocado, seed removed and cut into pieces
1/2 punnet grape tomatoes, cut into halves
1/4 purple cabbage, grated
1 bunch fresh coriander, chopped
1/2 bunch fresh mint, chopped

I combine all the green ingredients into a salad serving bowl and gently fold through the avocado.
To decorate I use the grape tomato halves, placing them around the outside of the bowl with the pomegranate seeds in the centre. I like to get a bit fancy where I can with my presentation! Pour over a generous drizzle of olive oil and a squeeze of fresh lemon with a pinch of cracked pepper. Enjoy this salad experience, it sure will satisfy!

Balsamic, Feta and Cos Lettuce Salad

I absolutely love the textures and flavours in this salad. This salad tastes great with freshly grilled tofu, oven roasted almonds or fresh grilled fish, and also pairs well with organic grilled chicken pieces , taking care to ensure where your poultry source has come from.

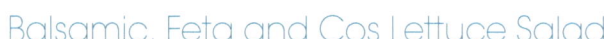

1 large handful fresh rocket
1 red capsicum, chopped into medium-sized pieces
1 cos lettuce, torn into rough pieces
1/2 bunch fresh mint, chopped
100g goat's cheese, broken into pieces (or add chosen form of protein - tofu, almonds, fish)

Arrange all ingredients onto a serving plate then dress with:
1 drizzle organic balsamic vinegar
1 drizzle olive oil
1 pinch cracked black pepper
1 squeeze fresh lime

Vietnam on a plate

I fell in love with the street food in beautiful Vietnam. The fresh, crisp flavours of chilli and mint combined with numerous authentic sauces.

2 Lebanese cucumbers, spiralized
1 handful fresh bean sprouts
1 red chilli, chopped
1 lime, cut into wedges (use as garnish as well as a fresh squeeze for the finishing touch)
1/2 cup raw peanuts, oven roasted on high for seven minutes, then roughly crushed
1 drizzle sesame oil
1 handful fresh mint, finely chopped
1 tbsp dried onion flakes

Arrange spiralized cucumbers on a serving platter, place fresh bean sprouts on top, then the chopped red chilli and fresh mint. Sprinkle over the crushed roasted peanuts and dried onion flakes, and finish with a drizzle of sesame oil and a generous squeeze of fresh lime.
Options: sweet and spicy chilli sauce or my coriander lime chilli dressing (see page 50) are also great flavours to add to this salad depending on personal taste.

Watercress, Cucumber and Spring Water Tuna Salad

After a workout, or even if I'm at a point where I'm just not sure what to eat, I often turn to this salad because it has so much to offer nutritionally. This recipe was a constant rescue for me in my hunger 'hour of need'. Being quite simple to create it is definitely a salad I recommend for a busy lifestyle, or for that moment when hunger hits. I eat this salad with pieces of tofu instead of tuna.

1 bunch fresh watercress, chopped
1/2 punnet cherry tomatoes
1 ripe avocado, seed removed and cut into slices
250g fresh tuna chunks or tuna in spring water or tofu
1 fresh lemon, juiced
1 pinch Himalayan salt
1 pinch cracked black pepper
1 drizzle olive oil

Or for dressing options (see dressings, sauces and dips page 47) Combine all ingredients, place on a serving plate and enjoy!

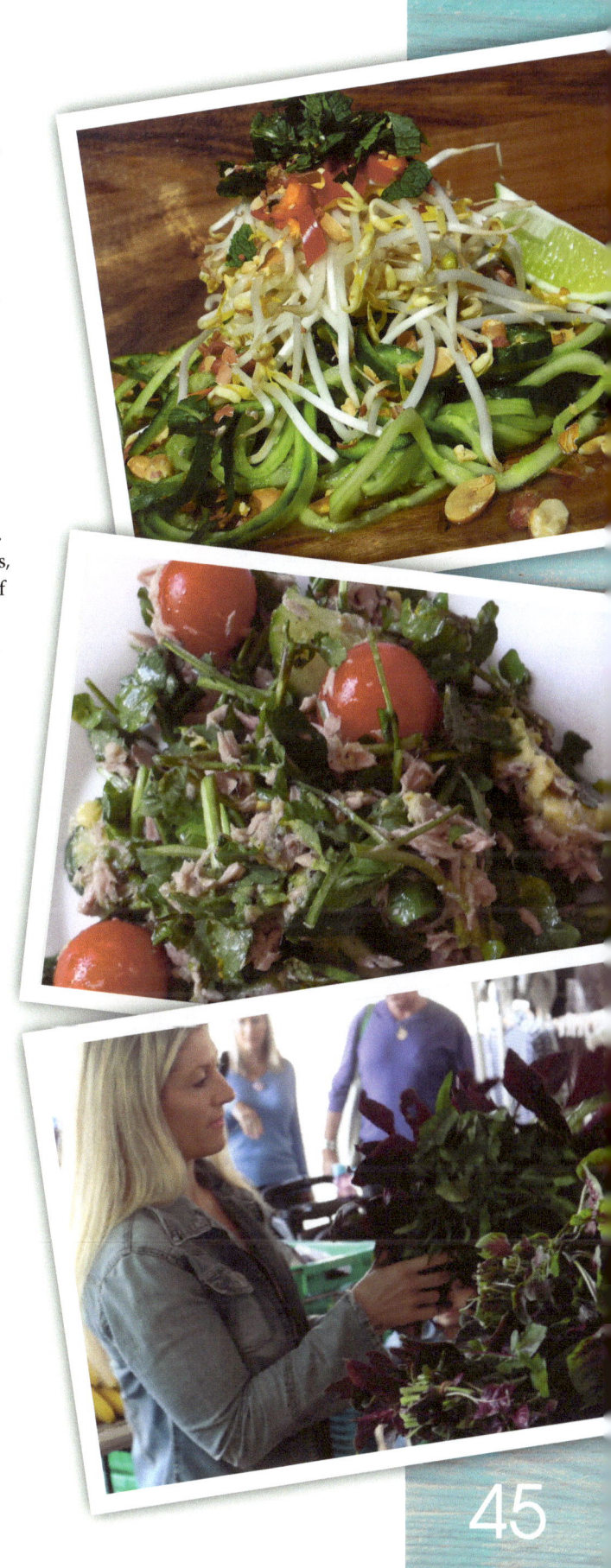

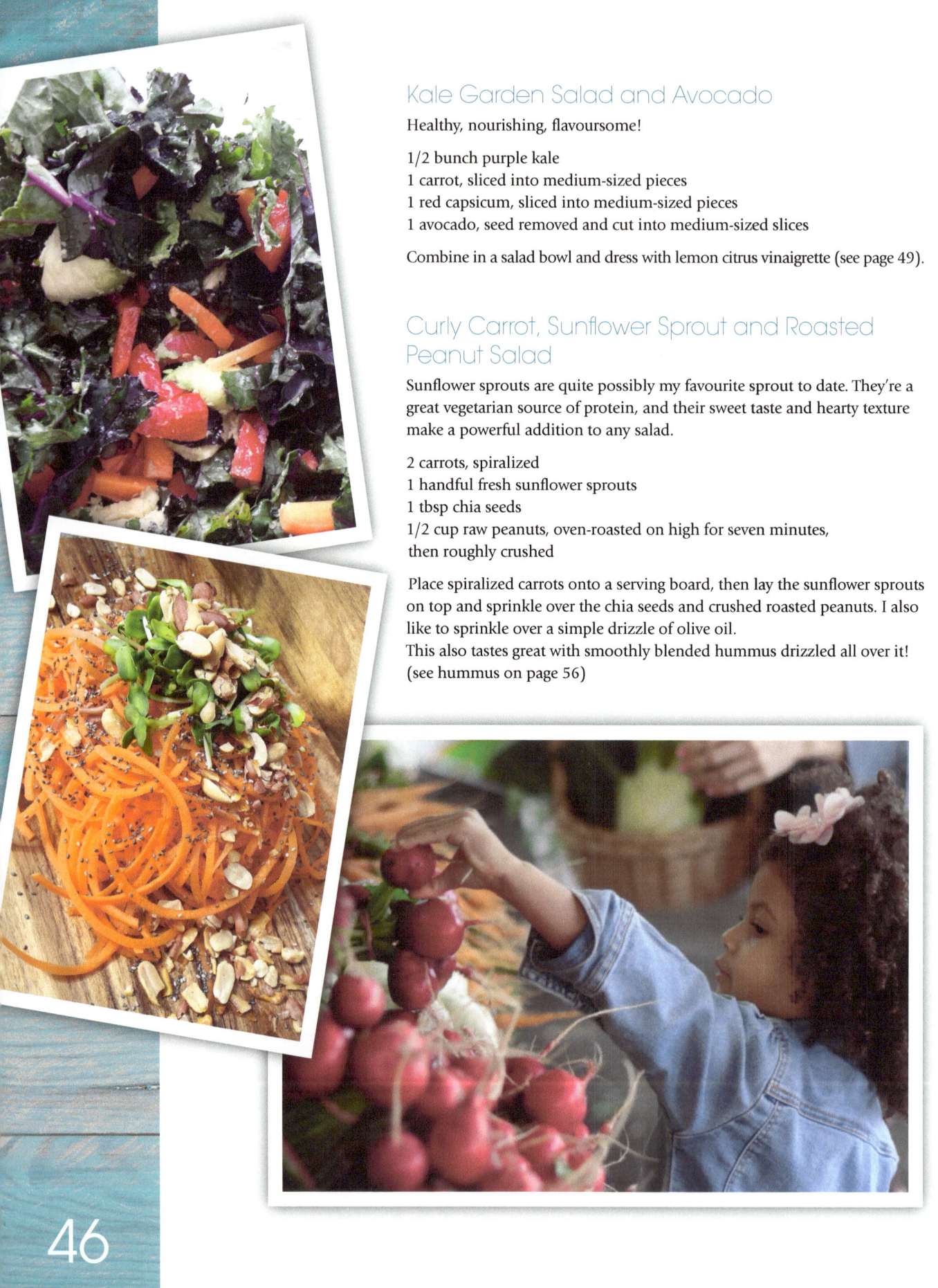

Kale Garden Salad and Avocado

Healthy, nourishing, flavoursome!

1/2 bunch purple kale
1 carrot, sliced into medium-sized pieces
1 red capsicum, sliced into medium-sized pieces
1 avocado, seed removed and cut into medium-sized slices

Combine in a salad bowl and dress with lemon citrus vinaigrette (see page 49).

Curly Carrot, Sunflower Sprout and Roasted Peanut Salad

Sunflower sprouts are quite possibly my favourite sprout to date. They're a great vegetarian source of protein, and their sweet taste and hearty texture make a powerful addition to any salad.

2 carrots, spiralized
1 handful fresh sunflower sprouts
1 tbsp chia seeds
1/2 cup raw peanuts, oven-roasted on high for seven minutes, then roughly crushed

Place spiralized carrots onto a serving board, then lay the sunflower sprouts on top and sprinkle over the chia seeds and crushed roasted peanuts. I also like to sprinkle over a simple drizzle of olive oil.
This also tastes great with smoothly blended hummus drizzled all over it!
(see hummus on page 56)

Adore Dips, Dressings and Sauces

I use farm fresh, natural organic ingredients in my sauces, dressings and dips. For me, a real dressing, sauce or dip is at its best when it's made from nature itself, not tampered with by chemicals, emulsifiers, additives, preservatives, or any other health destroying particle. It's amazing how nature literally has everything in it that our bodies truly need to sustain us and maintain health.

Often I make large amounts of my sauces and dressings so I have them on hand in my fridge in glass jars, lasting up to a few weeks. There is always a different flavour I can conveniently find in my home to add to my meals and salads. I just take out the jar of choice, give it a shake and pour it happily over my meal.

I tend to stick to using mostly olive oil, Himalayan pink salt, cracked black pepper and fresh lemon as a base for my dressings (see page 77 in herbs about lemon). The flavour is delicious mixed over salads, plus it's so good for you. Explore the flavours of fresh and natural, they're endless!

Guacamole

Guacamole adds amazing flavour and texture to many meals and snacks. I often eat avocado of a morning, or even create my guacamole or my smashed avocado (see page 49) to use as a spread. Avocado is great to use for thickening smoothies (see page 17 avocado smoothie) and I even use it as a yoghurt alternative (see page 21 avocado muesli). It tastes delicious, contains good fat that the body thrives on, and is loaded with important nutrients. This is how I like to create my own guacamole:

I blend the following ingredients together -
2 ripe avocados
1 small onion
2 cloves of garlic, peeled
1 pinch pink Himalayan salt
1 pinch cracked black pepper
1 red chilli (optional) stalk top removed
1 small green capsicum, stalk, seeds and ribs removed
1 small bunch coriander, only remove the roots and use the stalks as they have heaps of flavour
1 fresh lemon, skin and seeds removed
1 generous drizzle of olive oil

Optional extras I like to use: I personally love to add a handful of fresh mint leaves, a handful of fresh Italian parsley, and a thumb of fresh ginger for a hit of zing in my guacamole. Enjoy!

Creamy Cashew Dressing:

I like to use this dressing with many of my inspired Thai or Vietnamese recipes , especially with some of my salads that have an Asian influence, and in particular my Raw Pad Thai (see page 33).

I combine all of the following delicious ingredients into a high powered blender and blend until thick, smooth and creamy

1 orange, skin and seeds removed
1 crunchy red apple, cut it into quarters to assist with blending
1 large tomato, cut in half to assist with blending
1 bunch fresh coriander
3 cups raw cashews, soaked for 20 minutes or until soft
1 large lemon and 1 lime, skin and seeds removed
1 pinch Himalayan salt
1 generous pinch paprika
1 tbsp tamari
1 very generous drizzle olive oil

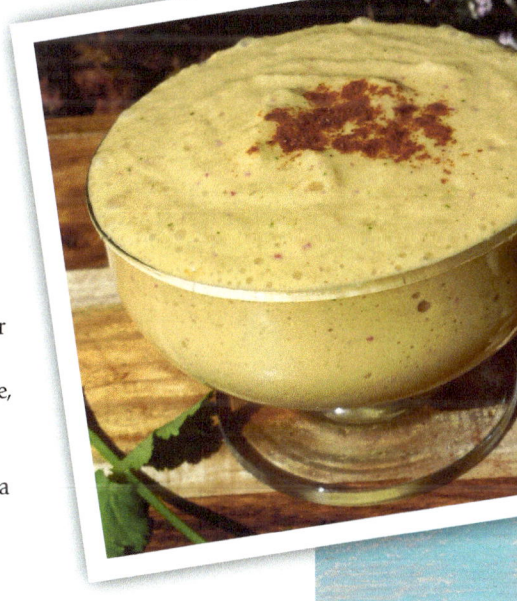

African Inspired Hot Chilli Dipping Sauce

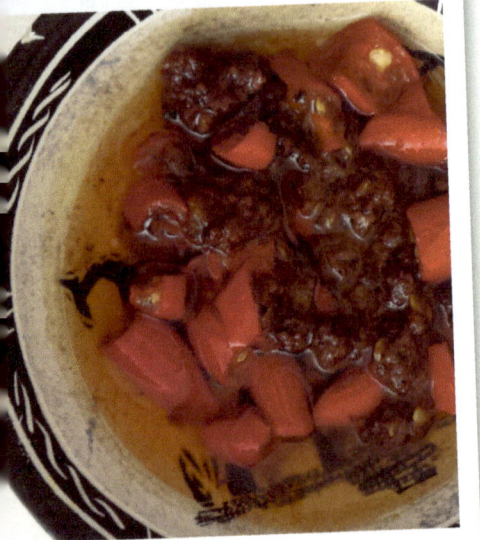

I can't get enough of the unique flavours of beautiful Africa. This sauce is a touch of Africa embracing hot spice. If you have just cooked and fried up onions, mushrooms or even an appropriately sourced steak, in coconut oil of course, and are about to throw that dirty pan into the sink to give it a good scrub, try making this sauce first before you do so.
Yes, straight after you have been cooking your chosen ingredient in your hot frying pan with coconut oil, add the following ingredients for my hot chilli dipping sauce into the used pan. Mix it all together, allowing it to cook for several minutes.

6 small red chillies, chopped, remove stems but keep the seeds
1/2 cup raw, and cold-pressed organic coconut oil
1 pinch pink Himalayan salt
2 cloves garlic, peeled and chopped
1 thumb fresh ginger, finely chopped

Mix all together with a spoon in a bowl then add to that "used" hot fry pan.
The flavours that are left in the pan, once the onions, mushroom or steak has been removed, combined with the ingredients of my hot chilli dipping sauce, add a delicious unique flavour to the finished hot chilli dipping sauce.
Place the sauce in a dipping bowl and enjoy. I like to eat my hot chilli dipping sauce with my homemade sweet potato wedges, yam or kumara fries (see page 55).
After all, I am a huge lover of chilli and it's a huge lover of me.
Note: as another option, you can always pour out the mixture into a hot non stick sandwich press and leave it to cook for several minutes that way , if you haven't already been cooking with a fry pan.

Tahini

For making my own tahini, I roast 500g sesame seeds in a pre-heated oven at 150 degrees, for approximately five minutes, stirring occasionally until slightly golden brown. Keep a very close eye on it, they do burn very easily.
Allow to cool then add to a food processor or blender. Blend and grind, gradually adding pure organic olive oil as necessary until a paste is formed.
Place in a sealed glass jar and keep in the fridge for up to 2 or 3 weeks.
Tahini can also be added to the ingredients of hummus, but as you will see in my hummus recipe (see page 56) it's really up to you, I don't always include tahini when making my hummus. Get creative with your favourite flavours and see what you come up with.

* I have also used my own dried out herbs in the blending process of tahini to create a touch of difference. Try it for a different tahini experience. Dried rosemary and thyme in particular are my favourites to add.

Garlic Dipping Sauce

This is another fabulous dipping sauce to be enjoyed with homemade sweet potato wedges, or yam and kumara fries, or I love it as a sauce poured over coconut oil pan fried mushrooms or mixed in with a brown rice dish. I use it with so many meals and salads to liven things up, and it sure sets taste buds flying!

Soak 3 cups of cashews in purified water until soft, then blend together with:
3 garlic cloves, peeled
1 large fresh lemon, seeds and skin removed
1 pinch of Himalayan salt
1/2 cup of pure, fresh organic coconut cream to taste
1 small onion, peeled
1 heaped tbsp of raw, cold-pressed organic coconut oil (or 2 tbsp if in liquid state)

Optional extras: I use fresh herbs like parsley, coriander or mint. They go so well with this sauce, and even a thumb of fresh ginger in the blending process will work.

Lemon Citrus Vinaigrette

This is pure, simple goodness. I use:
The juice of 1 fresh lemon and its pulp
1 very generous drizzle olive oil
1 pinch pink Himalayan salt
1 drizzle raw apple cider vinegar
Gently stir all together and enjoy!

Easy Herb and Mustard Seed Dressing with Lime

My healthy herb and mustard seed dressing is created from my memories as a young child. I recall eating boiled potatoes with a mayonnaise style mustard seed dressing. This recipe was born from those memories – with a nutritional spin on them!

1 handful fresh dill, finely chopped
1 handful fresh thyme, finely chopped
1 handful fresh rosemary, finely chopped
1 tsp brown mustard seeds
1 tsp yellow mustard seeds
1 drizzle raw apple cider vinegar
1 large drizzle olive oil
1 lime, juiced and use its pulp

Stir all together and allow to sit for an hour before serving, stirring occasionally. This will allow all the flavours of the fresh herbs to combine and fuse together.

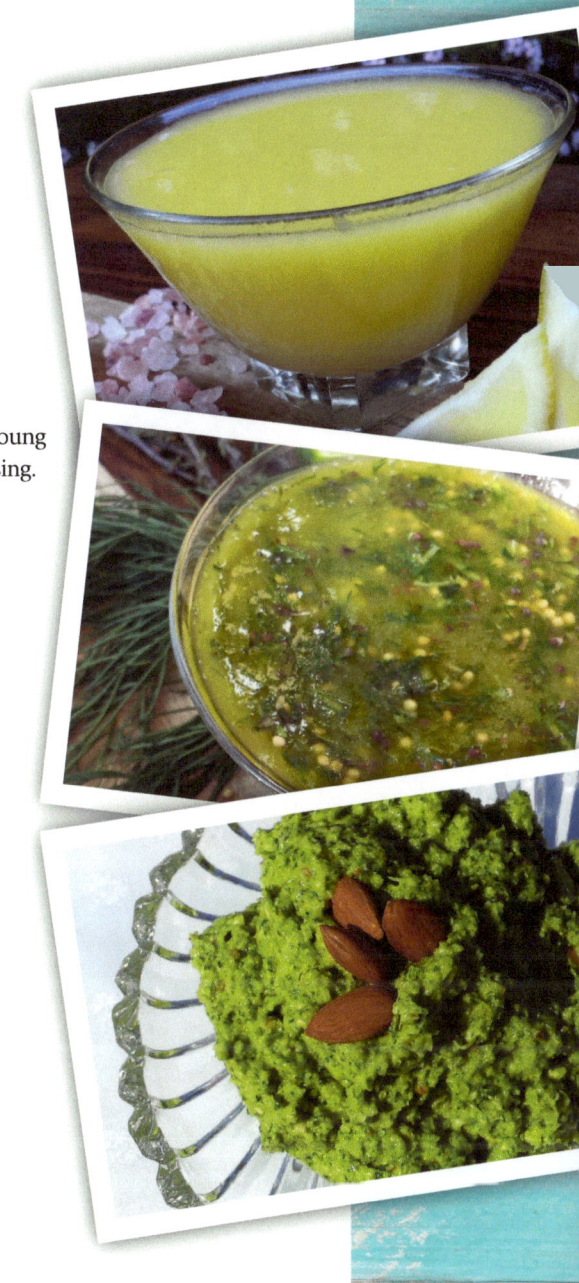

Pesto

I make my pesto by using all the stalks and stems that would otherwise be thrown out from fresh herb bunches and from fresh greens.

1 bunch coriander along with its stalks (of course) for added flavour
1 bunch spinach stalks
1 bunch broccoli stems
1 bunch kale stems
1 generous squeeze of fresh lemon juice
1 pinch Himalayan salt and cracked black pepper
1 generous drizzle olive oil,

Combine everything in a blender and mix until smooth.
Optional: you can add small amount, approx 2-3 capfuls, of raw apple cider vinegar.
Add a handful of raw almonds and the flesh of 1 ripe avocado (seed removed) to thicken up and create a delicious texture in the pesto. Pesto is ideal for a healthy snack or dip, or with grilled fish, fried mushrooms, grilled organic chicken or appropriately sourced steak.

Smashed Avocado

This is one of my all time favourite and super simple flavours that goes with so much!
All I do is mash 2 ripe avocados with the juice of 1/2 a large fresh lemon and a pinch of Himalayan salt. It's so easy to make. It's great as a side with a main meal or as a dip, and fabulous as a spread alternative to butter. Check out my smashed avocado and jacket kumara (see page 25). You've got to try it, I just love this!

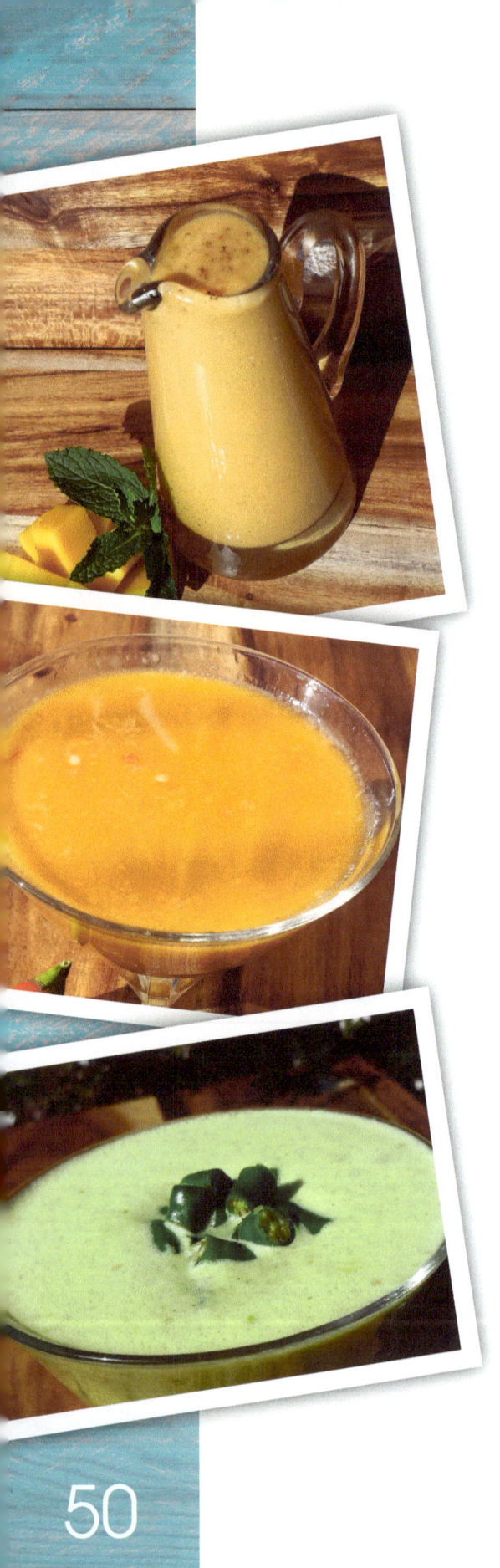

Mango and Pomegranate Dressing

This is great to have over salads, fresh fruit desserts, and also delicious as a creamy fruity pasta sauce too.

Flesh of 1 large ripe mango
seeds of 1 fresh pomegranate
1 cup pure, fresh, organic coconut cream
1 sprinkle coconut sugar to taste
1 sprinkle organic cinnamon

Blend all together until smooth.
Add into the blended mix 1 handful of freshly chopped mint leaves (optional) stir and enjoy!

Sweet and Spicy Chilli Sauce

This is my version of sweet chilli sauce – with a healthy twist.

For creating this sauce I use:
3 red chillies, stalks removed
1 generous drizzle coconut syrup
1 pinch Himalayan salt
1 cap full macadamia oil or avocado oil (optional: add 1 small tsp sesame oil)
1 fresh lime or lemon, skin and seeds removed
1/2 cup organic olive oil or melted raw cold-pressed organic coconut oil

Simply blend together until smooth and enjoy!

Coriander Lime Chilli Dressing

I like to make this in my mini chopper, but of course a blender will do the job just fine too. I enjoy this dressing with my 'Vietnam on a plate' salad (see page 45).

1 bunch fresh coriander
1 fresh lime, skin and seeds removed
1 dash of balsamic vinegar
1 dash tamari
1 pinch Himalayan salt
1 generous drizzle olive oil
1 fresh green or red chilli

Blend all together until smooth.

Fresh Tomato and Bay leaf Sauce

I absolutely adore the sweet aroma of bay leaves. Sometimes I cook chunky vegetable soups and various other hearty dishes with bay leaves, and it creates so much more of a divine flavour. Knowing that bay leaves assist the body in so many ways, particularly with hair health, heart health, anxiety and stress, as well as helping eliminate bad cholesterol, I just had to create a sauce using this incredible leaf. My fresh tomato and bay leaf sauce helps give that elegant touch of flavour to meals. I especially love to use this sauce with my plantain skewers (see page 34). This is what you will need to create it:

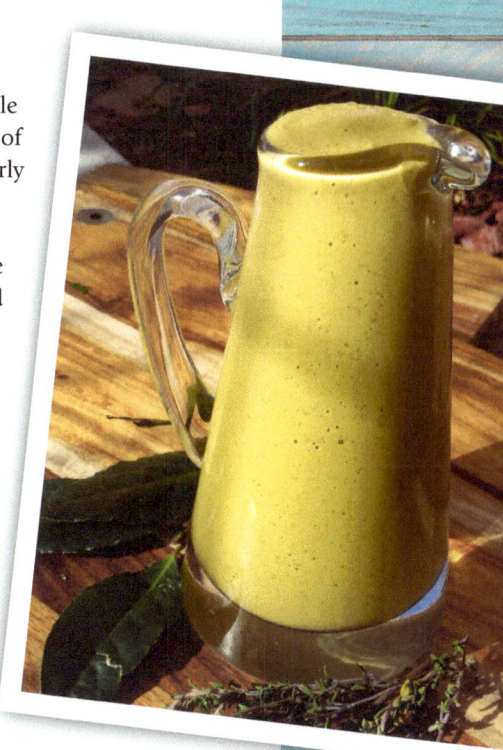

2 ripe tomatoes
1 large garlic clove, peeled
1 drizzle olive oil
1 small purple onion, outer skin removed
1 pinch Himalayan salt
1 fresh lemon, skin removed
1 generous handful fresh thyme
1 handful fresh Italian parsley or coriander

Blend together well until thick and smooth, then pour blended mixture into a glass jar adding 3 bay leaves.
Break each bay leaf in half to allow more aroma and flavour to be released. Seal the glass jar and leave in a cool shaded spot in the kitchen for around 3 hours, stirring occasionally, until all the flavours and aromas have combined. Keep stored in fridge.

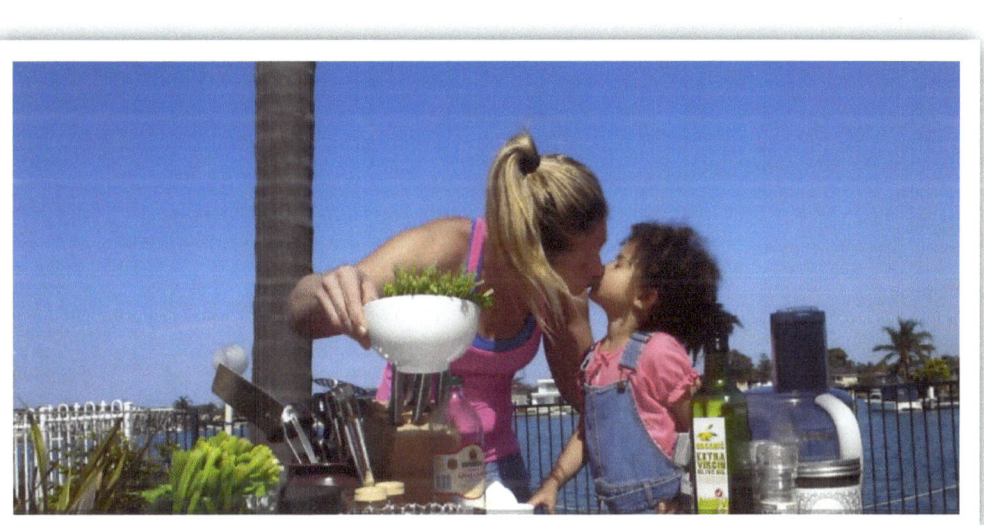

Reach for the foods that love your body and that your body will love.

Adore Snacks and Starters

When I think of snack time I get excited. I love experimenting with my many snack creations to satisfy hunger hits in the most natural and nourishing way possible! Little pieces of guilt-free pleasure straight from nature are what my snacks are all about. Eating the right kind of snack is very important for assisting energy levels and avoiding processed, refined sugars and harmful fats, or chemicals we are often unaware of in our food. Here is a taste of some of my delicious snacks and starters that I love to have on hand for maintaining a lifestyle of health and wellness.

Fruit Sticks

The vibrant colours alone make fruit so inviting, they make me just want to dive in and eat it! I absolutely love fruit! Fruit sticks are a superb way to make eating fruit exciting. I often use different kinds of fruit when I create these fruit sticks, but here I have used kumquats and strawberries together because the sweet and sour flavours compliment each other very well. They look super inviting too, and kids tend to go for inviting bright colours. Fruit sticks are great after school snacks, an awesome party pleaser, or perfect for that family picnic outing. All you will need is a bag of bamboo skewers and fruit of your choice – create away!

Power and Energy Balls

After making a delicious green juice, fruit juice or even a sweet carrot juice (see juice recipes page 13) there is lovely pulp left over! This is ideal to use to create delicious, nutritious snacks for kids' lunch box treats, movie nibbles, adventure outings, picnics, beach days – you name it! It's also a great way to reduce unnecessary waste! I create my power and energy balls straight from my juice pulp. I blend it all up so the pulp is of a smoother texture and add all sorts of scrumptious extra goodness to it to create my desired taste. Dates, raw honey, coconut sugar or syrup, figs to sweeten and raw cacao, nut milks, raw nuts, coconut, chia seeds, pepitas, goji berries, inca berries, or anything else that tickles my fancy that I might have in my kitchen. They all contribute to the exploding tastes and goodness in my power and energy balls.

They make for the perfect snack on the run too. I carry a few in a small container in my bag to devour when I'm out and about and hunger hits. It's also a fabulous way of avoiding junk food.

Carrot, Ginger and Walnut Energy Balls

Take the pulp from a delicious carrot juice (see page 15) and blend it in a high-powered blender until smooth, adding 1 large handful of raw walnuts. Roll into balls and enjoy.

Other optional ingredients to add: handful of fresh pineapple pieces, 6 pitted medjool dates, 1 scoop plant-based vanilla protein powder, coconut or a sprinkle of cinnamon.

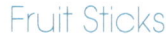

Green Power Energy Balls

Take the pulp from a delicious green machine juice (see juices page 14) and blend it in a high-powered blender until smooth, adding 1 large handful of raw almonds. Roll into balls. Enjoy!
Other optional ingredients to add: handful of organic dried figs or medjool dates to sweeten, 1 small scoop barley grass or wheat grass powder, coconut, 1 drop pure peppermint essential oil. Energy and Power Balls will keep in sealed container in fridge for 4-5 days.

Apple Peanut Stacks

My daughter loves the crunch of apples! Her excitement at watching peanuts being crushed into peanut butter is just priceless too. My apple peanut stacks came about one afternoon when my daughter asked me to make her a sweet treat. We all know kids don't have a great track record for patience when their hungry tummies are telling them to eat, so this quick and easy stack was created to satisfy the call of hunger within seconds. The perfect thing about these apple peanut stacks is that they are awesome for any occasion and for all age groups. Yes, the kiddies will get stuck into them but they are also a fabulous party entertainer and great for serving as appetisers.

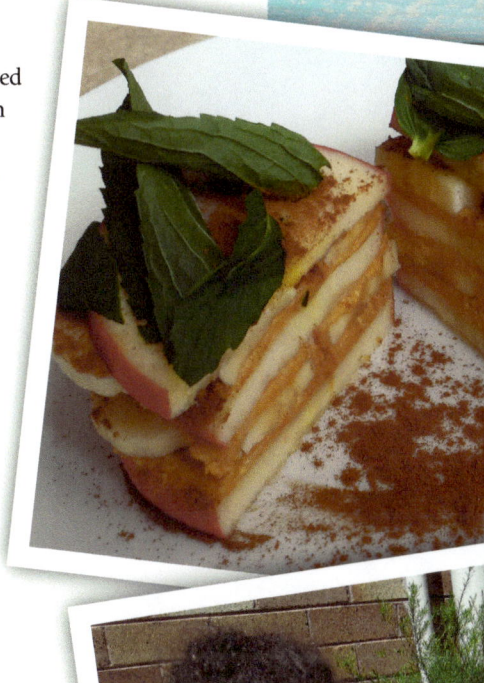

*Other nut butters, pumpkin, sesame, and sunflower spreads can be used as alternatives to organic peanut butter.

1 fresh, crunchy red apple
1 ripe banana
Organic cinnamon
Real, pure crushed organic peanut butter

Cut the apple in half and slice into thin, half-moon shaped slices.
Spread peanut butter over the first half-moon apple slice and sprinkle with cinnamon.
Slice the banana into pieces and then place 2 slices of the banana on top of the peanut butter and cinnamon.
Spread more peanut butter over the banana slices and add another apple slice on top. Repeat the process again and then place another apple piece on top to finish so each stack has at least 3 pieces of the apple slices layered.
Sprinkle organic cinnamon over each layer as you stack. Garnish with fresh mint leaves, enjoy!

Pineapple Paradise Slushie

This is so easy and so delicious it's ridiculous!

My daughter and I often whip up a Pineapple Paradise Slushie on a hot Summer day when a real thirst quencher is needed. Even in the cold months of the year we eat and drink fresh pineapple pieces and pineapple juice – it's ideal for coughs and colds, building strong bones and reducing stress. I mean, who doesn't feel great after eating a deliciously sweet ripe pineapple?

Remove the top of 1 pineapple.
With a sharp knife, slice down into the sides of the pineapple carefully between the skin and the flesh in a clockwise movement until the whole inside of the pineapple comes away. Take care not to push the knife through the bottom of the pineapple. Blend the removed pineapple flesh with ice cubes or previously prepared freshly frozen pineapple pieces. Pour the blended mixture back into the hollowed out pineapple, add a drinking straw and enjoy the precious taste of paradise! Optional extras to add into blended mix: handful fresh mint leaves, fresh mango, or fresh passion fruit.

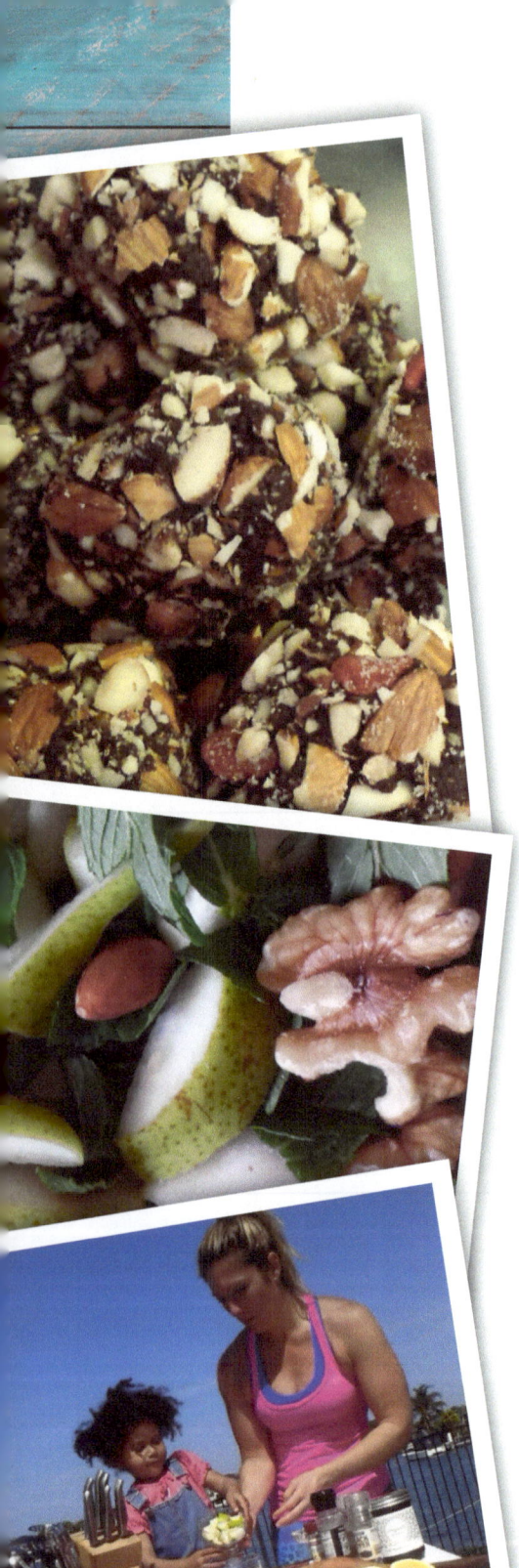

Raw Dark Choc Fruit and Nut Protein Balls

This recipe is my little treat of nourishing goodness and delight, stamping out those sweet cravings! Great for a snack on the run, lunch box treats, entertaining guests or simply enjoy with a much needed herbal tea (see page 74) of an afternoon

1 handful raw almonds
1 handful raw walnuts
1 handful raw macadamia nuts
2 tbsp chia seeds
1 cup cold organic green tea (prepared earlier)
4 heaped tbsp raw cold pressed organic coconut oil (or 8 if coconut oil is in liquid state)
1 cup cacao powder
1/2 cup goji berries

Optional extras: 8 pitted medjool dates for a sweeter taste, 1 handful raw cacao beans, coconut flakes

With these dark choc fruit and nut protein balls, I like to add as much or as little of each ingredient, according to my desired tastes and individual fitness or nutrition goals. That's the beauty of these raw treats, you don't have to worry about feeling guilty in the slightest. For me it's about keeping the fit in fitness, so I eat according to goals.
Roughly blend the walnuts, almonds, macadamia nuts and chia seeds, just slightly so they are still on the chunky side, and if desired add raw cacao beans here as well.
In a bowl, add the goji berries and raw cacao powder, and mix together, adding the roughly blended nut mix.
Melt the coconut oil (if not already liquid) and mix through the dry mixture. Add the cold green tea gradually, until the mixture is only ever so slightly gooey. Ensure the protein ball mixture is not too runny, and mix together well.
Crush or blend your choice of nuts or use coconut flakes with goji berries (rough blended mix of almonds with goji berries) and lay this out on a separate plate.
Create small ball shapes, then roll the balls over the crushed nut and goji berry mix.
Keep balls refrigerated in a sealed container for maximum freshness and enjoy, enjoy, enjoy!

Pear, Walnut and Mint Refresher

A quick, healthy and satisfying snack to have on the go, or to whip up for a healthy hunger hit at home. It's even a great dessert if eaten with fresh medjool dates and a dollop of organic greek yoghurt or a sprinkle of goat's cheese.

1 ripe pear, chopped into pieces
1 handful raw walnuts
1 handful fresh mint leaves, roughly chopped
Combine all three ingredients into a small serving bowl and enjoy.
Optional extras: goji berries, inca berries, fresh raspberries.

Sweet Potato Wedges, Yam and Kumara Fries with Garlic Dipping Sauce

These are one of my favourite quick snacks to whip up and indulge in guilt free. I often eat this of a mid-morning to boost my energy levels and keep them on point throughout the day.

1 each of sweet potato, yam, or kumara

Wash well, and keep the skin on, do not peel (most of the goodness is directly under the skin and peeling removes all of that). Cut the sweet potato, yam, or kumara in half then cut the halves into thick slices. Place the slices onto a non-stick sandwich press or under a grill and cook on both sides until golden and crispy.
While the sweet potato, yam, or kumara are cooking, whip up some delicious garlic dipping sauce (see page 48).
When cooked, I like to place onto a large serving plate and sprinkle with a generous pinch of pink Himalayan salt and enjoy with my scrumptious garlic sauce!

Banana, Cacao nib and Peanut Bites

My daughter and I eat a lot of bananas and fresh, natural home-made peanut butter. I decided to create bite-size snack treats that reflect our love for these flavours. My banana, cacao nib and peanut bites really are a snack for any occasion and any time of day. Bananas hold so much goodness, and coupled with the creamy texture of freshly made scrumptious peanut butter and the surprise crunch of the raw cacao nibs, these bites tick all the boxes for a tasty wholesome snack.

2 ripe bananas
1 small tub fresh organic crushed peanut butter (you can make your own by whipping up peanuts in a blender till smooth)
1 sprinkle of cacao nibs

Peel and slice the bananas into even thumb-sized pieces. Place the pieces of banana onto serving board.
Spread a dollop of peanut butter onto each piece of banana.
Sprinkle cacao nibs on top of the peanut butter.
Enjoy these delicious, quick and easy tasty bites of goodness!
Note: nut butters or even tahini (see page 48) work well as an alternative to peanut butter.

Did you know, eating two bananas before a strenuous workout packs an energy punch and sustains your blood sugar? They also protect against muscle cramps during a workout, or night time leg cramps. Bananas are also great help to improve your mood.

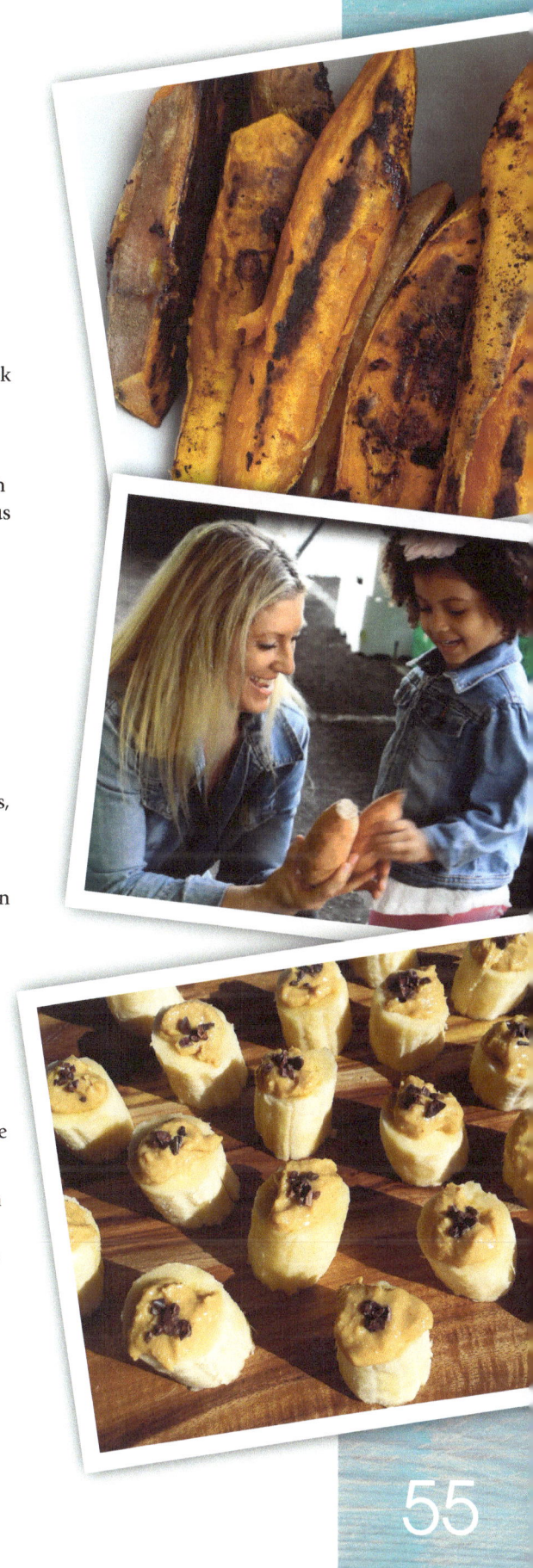

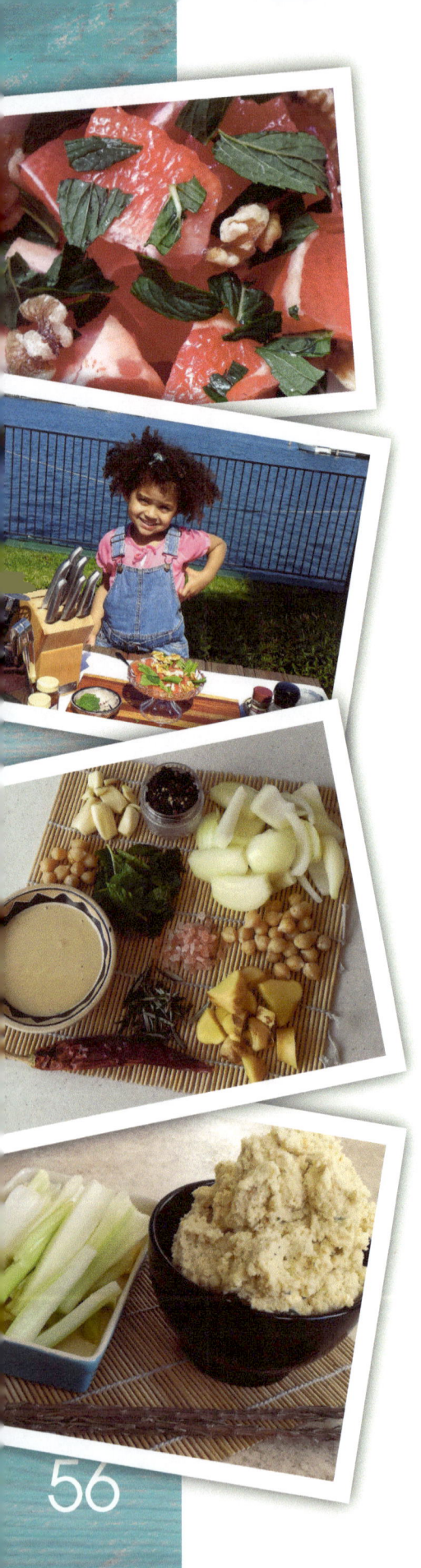

Red Grapefruit, Raw Macadamia and Mint Revitaliser

Grapefruit is amazing! It contains many vitamins, minerals and nutrients that our body needs for good health, plus it's super for boosting the metabolism. I find it a great food to help relieve stress, and it can even help fight gum disease. Red ruby grapefruit is definitely up there on my list of favourite fruits. Try this super easy revitaliser for a quick health-boosting snack.

1 whole chilled grapefruit, peeled and diced
1 handful raw macadamia nuts or raw walnuts
1 handful fresh mint leaves, roughly chopped
Combine all three ingredients in a small serving bowl and enjoy.
Optional extras: add freshly chopped strawberries, or fresh pomegranate.

Rosemary Mint Hummus

There's something so inviting about a hearty hummus dip. I'm sure you'll find this recipe as exciting as I did while I was creating the flavour. The fresh herbs I've included add that extra special zing to a much-loved dip.
Traditionally, hummus tends to be very smooth, which can easily be achieved with this recipe by thoroughly blending the ingredients to your desired texture, but I like to keep my hummus on the thick and fluffy side. That's the beauty of cooking – you create it ,you own it!

375g chickpeas
2 white onions, peeled and diced
4 cloves garlic, peeled
2 large thumb-sized pieces of fresh ginger
1 large handful fresh rosemary leaves
1 large handful fresh mint leaves
4 tbsp tahini, optional (can make your own see my recipe page 48)
2 large pinches Himalayan salt
3 large lemons, juiced
2 cups organic olive oil
1 red chilli (optional for added hot spice)

Soak the chickpeas in water overnight. Once soaked, rinse and boil for 45 minutes or until soft.
Place cooked chickpeas in a colander and rinse in cold water. Transfer to a blender and add the rest of the ingredients, except the olive oil and lemon juice. Blend the mix, adding olive oil and lemon juice gradually, until you have a smooth texture.
This dip is great to eat with any sort of vegetable dipping stick, such as carrot, celery, zucchini, broccoli, peppers or cucumber. Also delicious in cos lettuce, cabbage or Swiss chard wraps.
This hummus tastes amazing spread over warm sweet potato and sprinkled with fresh parsley, with my eggplant crisps (see page 61), or even in a small bowl topped with chopped up tomato, cucumber and dill, drizzled with fresh lime juice, olive oil and a sprinkle of paprika & cracked black pepper – delicious! Hummus really goes with so much and it's just so good for you!

Rainbow Veggie Sticks

This is the perfect way to make eating veggies fun and exciting for kids, or just to include as a healthy snack for a healthy lifestyle.

1 green capsicum, cut into small pieces
3 large Tuscan kale leaves, cut into rough pieces
1 purple beetroot, thinly sliced
1 large carrot, thinly sliced
1 zucchini, thinly sliced
1 golden beetroot, thinly sliced

Thread all sliced veggies onto skewers in alternating colours. Tastes great with my creamy cashew dressing (see page 47).
Note: I use my kitchen gadget graters (mentioned in my kitchen tools section see page 10) to make the thin slices for my rainbow veggie sticks.

Soft Raw Caramel Chews

A delicious health snack, and great to have stocked up in your freezer ready for any time of day! These chews are perfect for curing those last minute 'munchie' hits or sweet cravings.

500g raw cashews, soaked for 30 minutes or until soft in purified water
Blend the cashews on high speed with:
8 dried figs
3 heaped tbsp cacao nibs or cacao beans
4 heaped tbsp raw honeycomb or raw honey
1 generous drizzle of coconut syrup

Continue to blend until smooth.
Scoop the blended mixture onto a large sheet of baking paper. Place another sheet of baking paper over the top and press down, thinning the mixture out until it is like a flat sheet. Use a rolling pin if you have one. Place in freezer to set for 3 hours, or longer if possible.
Remove from the freezer, peel off top sheet of baking paper and cut into cubes or squares (or desired shapes). Place in an airtight container and keep stored in the freezer. Best eaten straight away from the freezer. Enjoy as a quick & easy snack while doing the house work, or for that afternoon treat with a delicious cup of organic herbal tea!

Tahini and Tomato Bites

These tiny tasty bites are full of flavour and goodness. I find more and more that it's the simple things that satisfy most. These bites satisfy any snack cravings .

1 punnet cherry tomatoes, halved
1 batch of tahini (see page 48)
1 large handful of freshly chopped Italian parsley
1 pinch cracked black pepper

Spread tahini over the tops of the sliced cherry tomatoes and arrange on a serving plate. Sprinkle over cracked black pepper and finely chopped Italian parsley. A squeeze of fresh lemon juice also tastes amazing on these tahini and tomato bites.

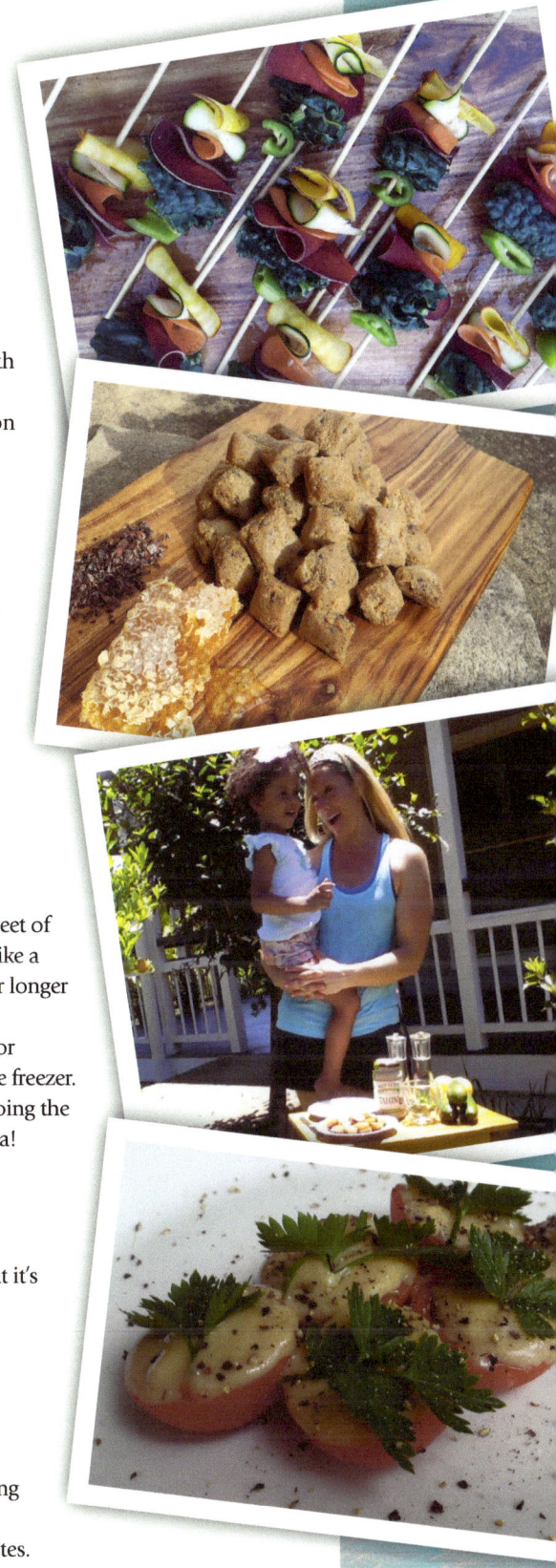

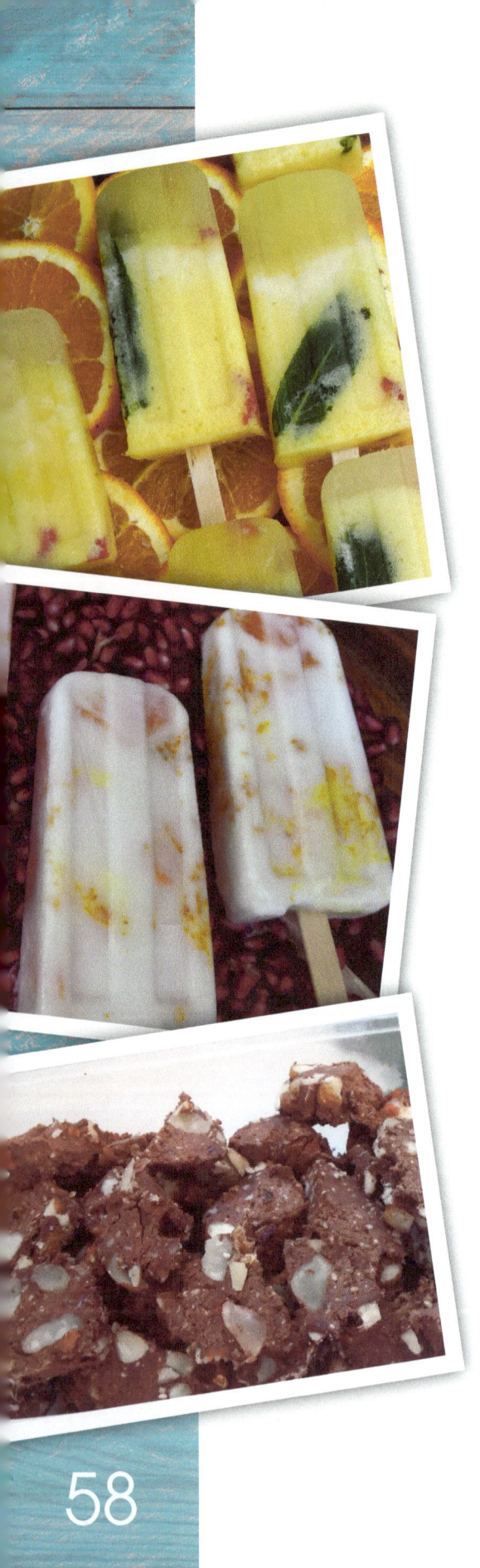

Pineapple, Chilli and Mint Ice Pops

I love the cool sweetness of pineapple against the hot and spicy hit of chilli in these thirst quenching ice pops. They're the perfect summer cooling treat.

1/2 fresh pineapple, blended until smooth
2 red chillies, seeds removed and chopped finely
1 handful fresh mint leaves

Pour the blended pineapple into ice pop moulds, adding pieces of chilli and mint leaves occasionally to splash the colour around.
Place in freezer for 3 hours. Enjoy!

Creamy Coconut, Tangerine and Turmeric Ice Lickers

This takes me back to my time in the tropics, my coconut filled days under palm trees – bliss! Combined with sweet tangerine and health-boosting turmeric, all those moments of joy are poured into this mouth-watering creation.

2 cups pure organic coconut cream
1 tangerine or mandarin , peeled and cut into small pieces
1 thumb-sized piece of fresh turmeric, grated

Pour coconut cream gradually into moulds, adding in each of the moulds pieces of tangerine or mandarin and fresh grated turmeric to the coconut cream to mix the flavours around and spread the colour through the ice blocks. Enjoy!
Note: if wanting a sweeter taste, blend pure coconut cream with 1 heaped tablespoon of coconut sugar before pouring into the moulds

Raw Rocky Road

Yes, that's right, healthy nourishing rocky road – you've got to try this recipe!

1 cup raw cacao powder
2 handfuls goji berries
1 handful raw almonds, roughly chopped
1 handful raw macadamia nuts, roughly chopped
6 heaped tbsp raw, cold-pressed coconut oil, or 12 tbsp if in its liquid state
1 handful raw brazil nuts, roughly chopped

With melted coconut oil, combine all ingredients together in a mixing bowl. Place mixture into a square or rectangular baking tray (lined with baking paper) and allow to set in the fridge for 5-10 minutes or until firm. Take tray out of the fridge and remove the set mixture, lifting it out with the baking paper. Place onto a cutting board and chop into chunks.
Keep refrigerated in a sealed container to enjoy when sweet cravings hit.
Note: for an even sweeter option add 6 pitted medjool dates and a generous drizzle of raw honey or even coconut syrup when mixing up your rocky road.

Mango and Rasperry Ice Blocks

The colour of these ice blocks are amazing, not to mention the combination of tastes, and they only take minutes to put together.

1 very ripe mango, blended well
1/2 punnet fresh organic raspberries

Pour the blended mango into moulds, adding fresh raspberries in each mould as desired. Place in the freezer for 3 hours , or until set. Enjoy!

Watermelon and Lychee Lickers or Passionfruit and Watermelon Ice Pops

These watermelon and lychee lickers are perfect to have on hand for a hot Summer's day – they're super healthy and absolutely delicious!

1/4 fresh watermelon, blended until smooth
1 handful lychees, cut into quarters, seeds removed
Carefully pour the watermelon into ice block moulds, adding lychee pieces in each. Place in freezer overnight, or until frozen. Enjoy!

For my Passionfruit & Watermelon Ice Pops:
1/4 fresh watermelon, blended until smooth
3 ripe passionfruit
Spoon passionfruit into ice block moulds, slowly adding the blended watermelon. Place in freezer overnight, or until frozen. Enjoy!

These ice pops are so sweet and delicious just the way they are. I often have these made up in my freezer as a great instant snack and frozen fruit treat. My daughter especially loves them!

Raw 'Cobana' Bombs

These delicious Raw 'Cobana' Bombs (coconut and banana balls) came about after I experienced an exceptional afternoon of cultural cooking with some amazing people I was privileged to meet in the unique villages of Fiji. The freshest coconut, the amazing texture and taste of real home grown fresh banana – all combined into an exploding bomb of bliss in your mouth.

3 very ripe bananas, mashed
6-8 pitted medjool dates, very finely chopped
1/2 cup organic activated plain buckinis
3 cups fresh-scraped coconut, (this fresh coconut is in the ideal moist state for making these 'cobana' bombs. You can always use desiccated coconut as an alternative, but you will need to add 1 cup of coconut oil to create the moist texture. I highly recommend taking the fresh-scraped option)

Reserve 1/4 cup of the scraped coconut on a plate. Mix the remaining ingredients together then roll into balls.
Roll the balls over the remaining 1/4 cup of scraped coconut.
Keep refrigerated in sealed container – they will last up to seven days, and are best eaten chilled from the fridge.
Options: add 1/2 cup crushed almonds or cashews into the mixture for a nuttier flavour, a generous organic cinnamon sprinkle and 1 cup of blended rolled oats or almond meal if looking for less of a moist texture.

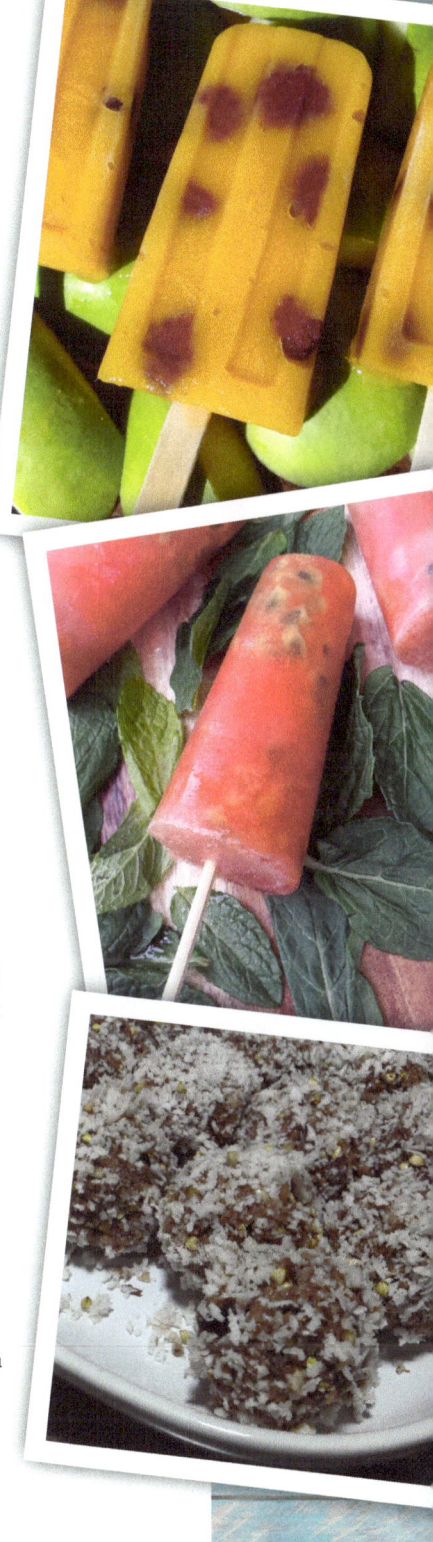

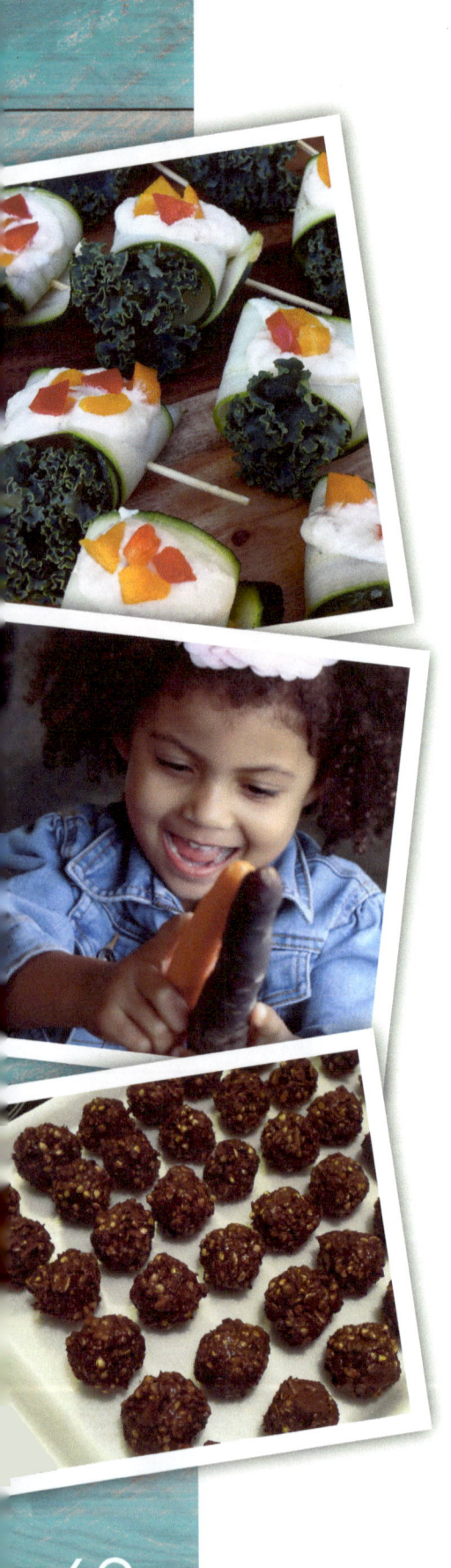

Zucchini Rolls with Creamy Pine Nut Cheese

The creamy pine nut cheese in this snack just makes it so scrumptious!

1 zucchini, thinly peeled into slices
1/2 punnet red and yellow tomatoes, or use red and yellow capsicums, finely diced
1 purple onion, finely diced (optional)

Pine nut cheese: 100g pine nuts, 1 sprinkle Himalayan salt, 1 dash purified water and 1 small lemon juiced. Blend together until thick, creamy and smooth.

Zucchini rolls: Place desired filling onto thin zucchini slices. I like to use curly kale but other options could be smashed avocado (see page 49), grilled chicken pieces appropriately sourced, fresh tuna or brown rice.
Gently roll and secure with toothpicks.
Spread pine nut cheese on top of the rolls and sprinkle over the tomatoes or capsicum, and purple onion if desired. You can even add fresh herbs like coriander on top of the pine nut cheese.

Another way you can try using this recipe –

Bruschetta Boats:

Spread a generous amount of pine nut cheese on top of zucchinis that have been cut in halves.
Place red and yellow tomatoes or capsicum, purple onion, and fresh herbs of your choice on top of the pine nut cheese.
Enjoy these delicious zucchini rolls or bruschetta boats!

Raw Choc Protein Balls

My nut-free, plant-based protein balls are oh so delicious and nutritious! Of course you could add crushed nuts of your choice if you wanted, it's entirely up to you. This is simply how I adore eating them.

1 cup shredded coconut
1/2 cup organic plain activated buckinis
3/4 cup raw cold-pressed organic coconut oil (in its liquid state)
1 generous drizzle of raw honey or coconut syrup to taste
1/2 cup raw cacao powder
1/4 cup chocolate plant-based protein powder
1/4 cup carob powder
1/4 cup coconut sugar (optional)
1/2 cup desiccated coconut
1 pinch pink Himalayan salt
1 generous sprinkle organic cinnamon

Combine all ingredients into a bowl and mix together.
Place in the fridge for 5-10 minutes or until the mixture has slightly hardened (this makes it easier to mould the mixture into balls) then take out of the fridge and stir again.
Making sure to have clean hands, shape the mix into balls.
Store in sealed container in the fridge and enjoy a delightful healthy guilt-free treat any time!

Snacks To Have On Hand

Instant and Amazing Snack – to Kick those sugar cravings

Freeze medjool dates as is – yes just as they are! I just remove the seed and cut each one in half, placing them in a sealed container in the freezer. They are a delicious sweet snack to eat straight from the freezer. Try it!

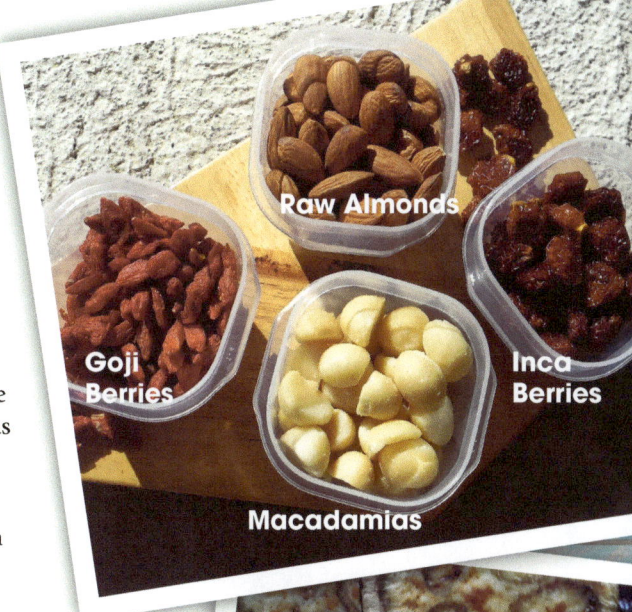

Toasted Garlic and Eggplant Crisps

Eggplant is a good source of dietary fibre and magnesium, just to name a few of its amazing benefits. I love finding new ways to create delicious dishes using eggplant. My toasted garlic and eggplant crisps are by far one of my favourite ways to enjoy eating this very versatile vegetable.

2 cloves garlic, skin on and gently squashed open by pressing down on them with the back of a spoon
1 eggplant, sliced into moderately thin slices

Place eggplant and squashed garlic cloves under a grill and drizzle all over with coconut oil. I like to spread coconut oil on both sides of the eggplant with a knife. Turn often until they are golden and crispy on both sides.
Place on serving plate. Sprinkle with Himalayan salt. Enjoy!

Nut Crunch Slice

I make a stack of my nut crunch slice and have it stored in my freezer for those emergency snack moments. It tastes like a naughty indulgence, but it's full of nourishing goodness, perfect for that much needed unwind after a busy day with a gorgeous soothing herbal turmeric tea (see page 76).

1/2 cup tahini (see page 48)
1/2 cup freshly-ground smooth organic peanut butter
1/4 cup raw honey
1/2 cup sesame seeds, roasted in hot pre-heated oven for 5min
1/2 cup pepitas, roasted in hot pre-heated oven for 7min
1/2 cup almonds, roasted in hot pre-heated oven for 7-9min

Combine tahini, peanut butter and raw honey together and mix well. Place the mixture onto a sheet of baking paper.
Sprinkle the sesame seeds, pepitas and almonds over the top of the mixture.
Place another sheet of baking paper on top of the mix and press down to flatten it all out, or alternatively use a rolling pin.
Place in the freezer to set for 2 hours or until firm.
Remove from the freezer when set, cut into slices when you're ready to eat and enjoy!
Keep stored in sealed container in the freezer, best eaten when very chilled straight from the freezer.

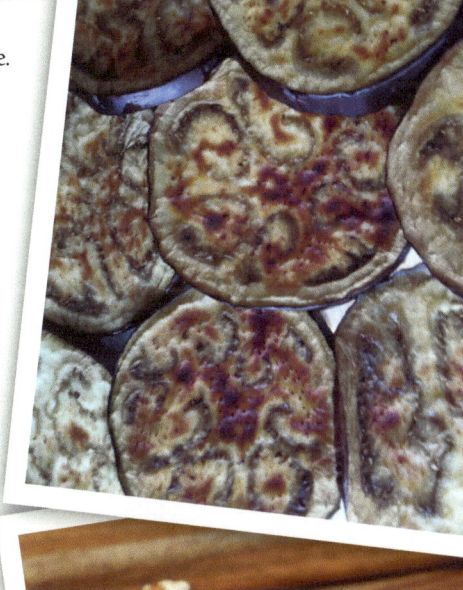

Adore Dessert

Many of my desserts are created around raw, plant-based eating. I don't use any refined sugars, sweeteners or dairy at all to achieve the tastes – there's simply no need. It's really just a matter of knowing how to use what nature provides, and how to extract the flavours, textures and tastes desired. Raw honey, raw honeycomb, medjool dates, coconut syrup, coconut sugar; these are just some of nature's amazing sweeteners. I love edible plants, they have a way of giving us exactly what we need, and if we use them to our advantage the creative possibilities are endless. Here are some desserts I absolutely love to savour, knowing all the while that guilt is never an issue. I am actually left feeling light and enriched after eating raw desserts. Healthy and nutritious dessert options? How awesome! It really is an exciting avenue to explore.

Here's a peek into my world of mostly raw, nourishing desserts and treats...

Red Ruby Sorbet

It doesn't get much better than this! I absolutely love red ruby grapefruit, it's only a tiny fraction on the sour side but it hits you with a surprise burst of sweetness at the same time, unlike yellow grapefruit that tends to come down more on the sour side. I have pre-prepared fresh fruit, cut and waiting in my freezer.

2 frozen red ruby grapefruit
1 punnet frozen strawberries
1/4 frozen watermelon
2 limes, freshly squeezed
1 cup purified water

Blend it all up, serve in a daiquiri style glass and enjoy this heavenly experience!

Strawberry Banana Delight Cream Bombs

These Banana bombs are such an easy, delicious dessert.

1 punnet strawberries, de-stalked, cut in half, frozen in zip lock bag
3 bananas, peeled, sliced into thick pieces, frozen in zip lock bag
4 heaped tbsp of raw, cold-pressed organic coconut oil or 8 tbsp if already in a liquid state
2 tbsp organic cacao powder

Add cacao powder to melted coconut oil and stir until smooth
Alternatively use carob powder or add plant-based choc protein powder for a lighter choc flavour.
Blend frozen bananas until thick and creamy (see banana delight cream recipe page 65).
Scoop banana mix onto the halved frozen strawberries with a teaspoon.
Drizzle with the cacao and coconut oil mixture until coated.
Place on a serving board and put back in freezer for three minutes to set.
Serve chilled and enjoy!

These treats can be kept in the freezer in an airtight container for up to two weeks.

Raw Blueberry 'Ice-Cream' Cheesecake

This cake is such an easy satisfier – deliciously sweet goodness that you can indulge in any time of the day. I often make this raw 'cheesecake' at the beginning of the day, leaving the cake to set nicely in the freezer, serving it up for a surprise dessert. The fact that this cheesecake is made from raw ingredients will amaze any taster. It's a fabulous alternative for destroying sweet tooth cravings. Not only does it taste divine, it will last in the freezer for a few weeks, giving you instant dessert. It really is an awesome way to avoid reaching for processed sweets that will harm your body and health. You can add various flavours or spices to your desired tastes, but I like to make my raw blueberry cheesecake like this.

You will need a standard size spring form cake tin.

Base:
1 cup pitted medjool dates
1 cup dried figs
1 tbsp organic cinnamon
1 thumb-sized vanilla pod
1 cup raw hazelnuts
Blend all together to a thick paste, then spread out over cake tin base, pressing down firmly till even all over.

Filling:
1 cup fresh blueberries
4 large frozen bananas
Blend together till silky smooth and spread out on top of the base, then place cake tin in the freezer while preparing next element.
1 cup raw macadamias or 1 cup raw cashews
3 frozen bananas

Blend all together till silky smooth and layer this mixture on top of the previous layer.
Decorate cake top with blueberries, crushed raw hazelnuts and pistachios.
Keep cake in freezer to set for 4 hours.
Take out five minutes before ready to serve. Eat chilled. Enjoy!
Keep stored in the freezer in a sealed cake container.

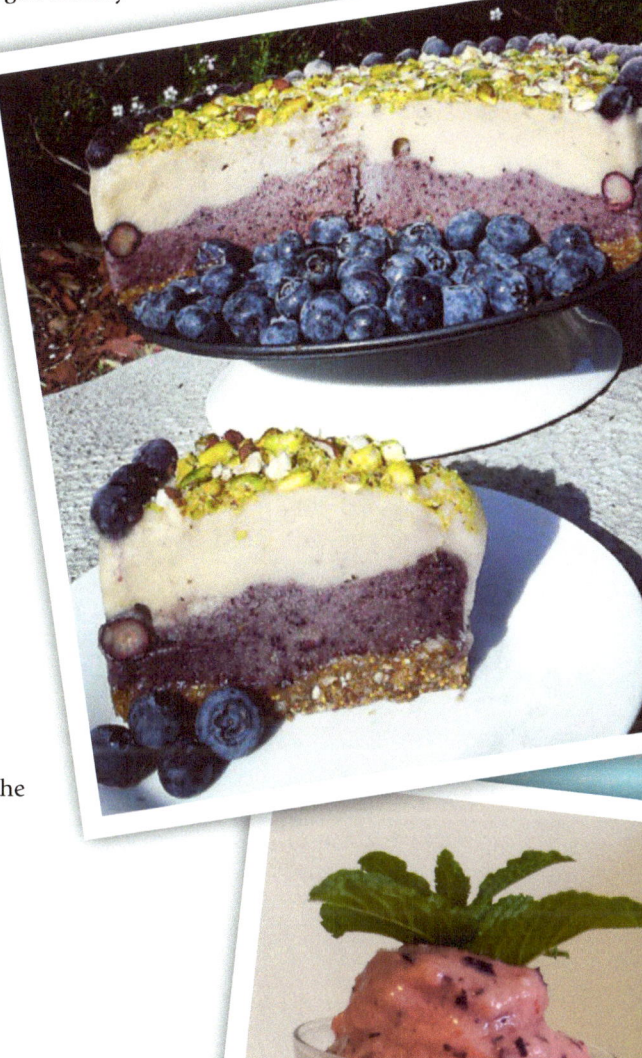

Plum Sorbet

I love the taste of this plum sorbet, it's soooo good! The kids will love this too, and won't even know how good it is for them!

8 ripe plums, de-seeded, halved and frozen in a zip-lock bag
1 cup almond milk (see recipe page 11) or 1 cup freshly made coconut milk (see page 11)

Blend the frozen plums and milk of your choice until smooth and creamy.
For optional flavour extras add 1 thumb-sized vanilla pod and 4 pitted medjool dates when blending for a sweeter taste.
Serve in a tall glass and garnish with fresh mint.
This is an amazing cooler in the heat of summer or as a special afternoon treat – even an energy booster to enjoy on the go!

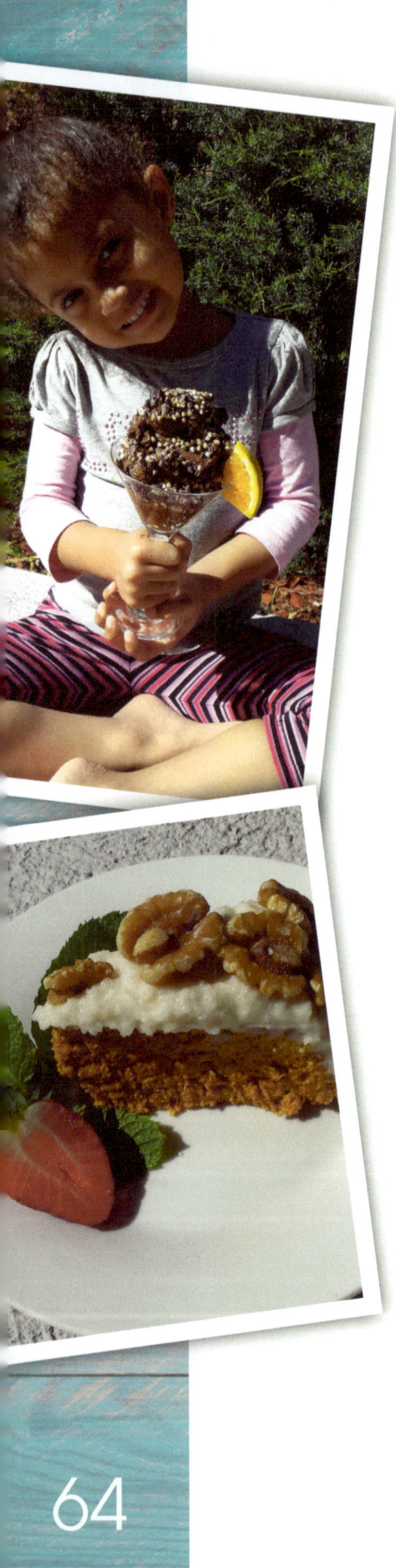

Raw Choc Crunch Mousse

Yes it really does taste like mousse, and the great thing about this recipe is how good all the ingredients are for you. Who would have thought you could indulge in scrumptious chocolate mousse guilt-free! Here is my version of Raw Choc Crunch Mousse to enjoy at your eating pleasure.

To a blender add:
3 ripe avocado
1/4 cup raw carob powder
1 generous sprinkle cinnamon
1/2 cup raw cacao powder
8 pitted medjool dates

Blend all ingredients together until silky smooth.
Place blended mixture into serving glasses and sprinkle with raw cacao nibs and organic activated plain buckinis. I also like to garnish with a slice of fresh orange.

Raw Carrot Cake

This Carrot cake ticks all the boxes for any cake craving. A cake that is healthy, nutritious and guilt-free? Yes please! I've created the foundation of this cake using the pulp of my carrot juice (see page 15) and my Pineapple, Lemon and Ginger juice (see page 16). It's very satisfying being able to transform remnants of food that might otherwise be thrown away into delicious and nutritious desserts.

In a high powered blender place:
Pulp from fresh carrot juice (see page 15)
Pulp from Pineapple, Lemon and Ginger juice (see page 16)
8 pitted medjool dates
1 very generous drizzle of raw honey
1 sprinkle organic cinnamon

Turn out blended mixture into a mixing bowl when smooth and add:
1 cup crushed raw walnuts, then gradually add:
1 – 1 1/2 cups of almond meal to thicken, stirring together.

The coconut pulp left over from making your own coconut milk (see page 11) also works really well in this recipe as an alternative to almond meal or do what I do – I sometimes include 1 cup of the coconut milk pulp here as well as the almond meal. When all ingredients are combined, place in a standard size spring form cake tin, pressing down firmly.

Icing:
1 1/2 cups raw macadamia nuts, blended with:
1 fresh lemon, juiced
1 pinch Himalayan salt

Then melt:
2 heaped tablespoons of raw and cold-pressed organic coconut oil,
or use 4 tablespoons if already in liquid form.
Mix all ingredients together in a blender until smooth and spread out on top of the cake. Decorate with crushed or whole raw walnuts and fresh strawberries and enjoy!
Will keep refrigerated in a sealed container for up to 5 days.

Cookie Dough

Who doesn't like to get stuck into a good lot of cookie dough, right? Especially a super healthy version! It's really easy and quick to whip this up, and it keeps well in the fridge for up to a week. Why not try this cookie dough for that late night movie snack?

3 cups almond meal
1/2 vanilla pod
2 tbsp vanilla plant-based protein powder
1 cup almond milk (see page 11)
1 generous sprinkle cinnamon
1/4 cup coconut sugar

Blend all ingredients together, gradually adding almond milk and being careful not to make mixture runny. Mixture should be like a thick dough.
Optional: add cacao nibs for an "oreo" tasting dough with a crunch after the mixture has been blended, or add 4 pitted medjool dates during the blending process for added sweetness.

Salty-Sweet Raw Banana Delight Cream

So simple, so delicious, so good!
Blend 3 frozen bananas until creamy, thick and smooth, and place blended mixture in a serving glass for plain banana delight cream.
I like to garnish my banana delight cream with crushed raw hazelnut pieces or cacao nibs.
For that salty-sweet flavour I add 1 generous pinch of pink Himalayan salt with the frozen bananas when I'm blending, along with 1 sprinkle of organic cinnamon. For extra sweetness I blend 4 pitted medjool dates in with the frozen banana.
I can never get enough of this guilt free goodness!

Licorice Delight Cream

I'm a real sucker for licorice. I just love it! This is a fun, healthy ice-cream option for someone like me who adores the taste of licorice! It's so easy, and you only need two ingredients to make it! Other flavour enhancing options can be used, like a sprinkle of cinnamon or a vanilla pod, but all I do is blend till powdery and as crushed as possible:

3 star anise
Add in 3 frozen bananas and continue blending ingredients till creamy and smooth. Serve in a tall glass – eat chilled and enjoy!

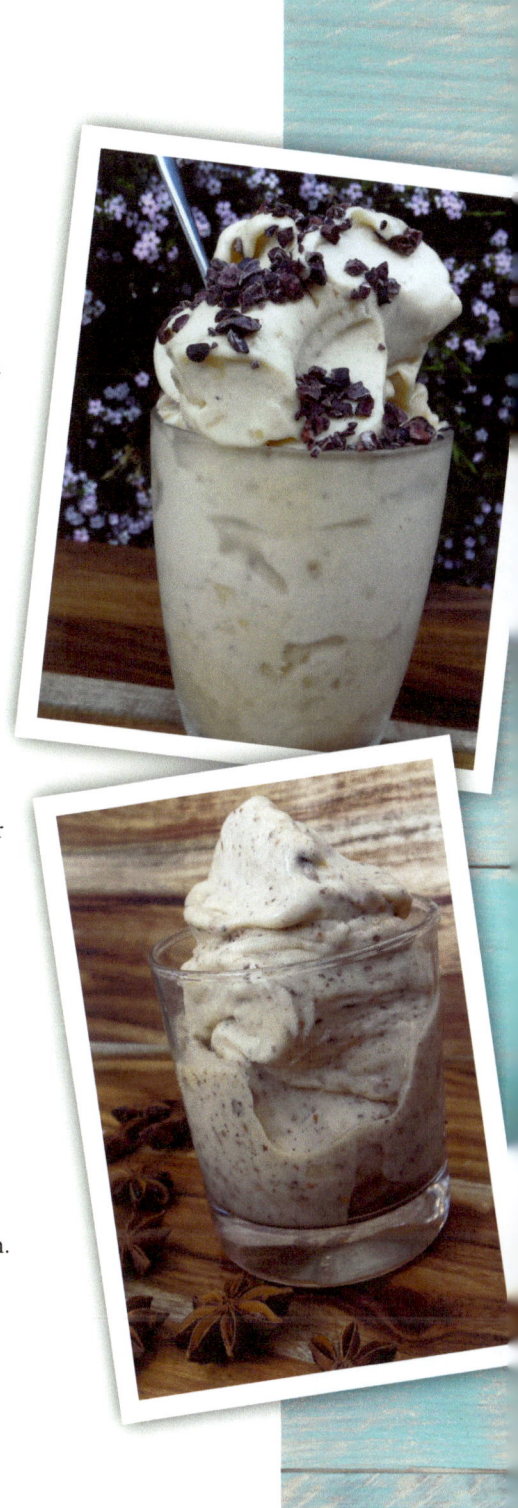

Results will come.

Persist. Persevere. Prevail!

Raw Strawberry Cheesecake

I eat a lot of fresh organic strawberries and also use them in many creations, mostly because they're nutrient-rich and packed with antioxidants. Strawberries have become a great friend of mine because they're known to help keep wrinkles at bay and aid in weight management. What a bonus! The gorgeous sweetness of strawberries is one of my favourite tastes and so a raw dessert straight from these delightful berries just has to be done.

I start by creating the base of my raw strawberry cheesecake.

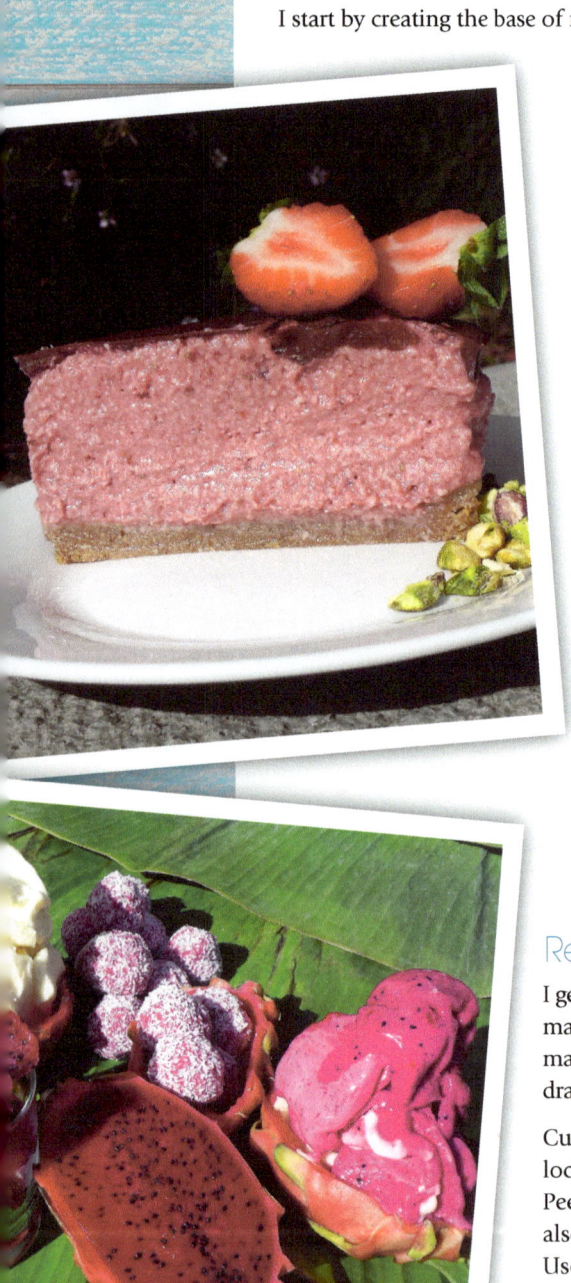

Base:
Combine 1/2 cup raw brazil nuts, 1/2 cup raw cashews, 6 pitted medjool dates, 1 drizzle of purified water and blend well together.
Place combined base in a small spring-form cake tin, firmly press down to make sure the base is compact in the tin. I often have enough mixture to make a few cakes in small tins.

Filling:
Wash, remove stems and then blend 1 punnet of strawberries with 8 pitted medjool dates and 2 scoops of vanilla plant protein powder, then add:
1/2 cup raw macadamias and continue to blend along with:
1 1/2 cups desiccated coconut.
If the filling is too moist add more desiccated coconut until the desired texture is reached, or add 3/4 cup of organic virgin cacao butter instead of extra desiccated coconut – melt it and blend it through the mixture. This will help to gently firm up the filling.
Spread filling on top of the base.

Topping:
Melt and mix 3 heaped tablespoons of raw, cold-pressed organic coconut oil (or 6 tablespoons if in its liquid state), with 1 heaped tablespoon of raw cacao powder and drizzle over the top of the filling already in the cake tin.
Place in freezer for 15 minutes or until set. Leaving in freezer longer will also help set the filling better.
Remove from freezer and from the tin when ready to serve. I like to add the finishing touch and decorate with fresh strawberries and crushed raw pistachios. Eat chilled, enjoy!

Red Dragon Fruit Delight Cream

I get so excited by this incredible exotic fruit, especially its brilliance in colour! It makes for sensational fresh fruit juices, smoothies and desserts, not only for its many health benefits, but its captivating colour is so inviting! (see page 77 for dragon fruit uses)

Cut 1 red dragon fruit in half and scoop out the flesh. Place the flesh in a zip lock bag and freeze overnight.
Peel 3 very ripe bananas and cut into pieces. Place pieces into zip lock bag and also freeze overnight.
Use a high-powered blender to blend the frozen dragon fruit flesh and banana pieces together until smooth and thick.
Eat as is, or add small amount of organic coconut cream or a dash of pure coconut milk while blending.
Instead of bananas, another great option is to use 1/2 a pineapple sliced into small pieces and frozen in zip lock bag. Blend with the dragon fruit and enjoy!

Dragon Fruit drink cubes

Mash red dragon fruit and place into ice-cube trays then pop into the freezer. These are great to add to fresh fruit juices for added texture, flavour and fabulous colour!

Raw Mint Choc Slice

I created this dessert with two things in mind – firstly to find a healthy option to choc mint slice, and secondly, I wanted to avoid throwing out and wasting the pulp from my gorgeous green juices. I came up with this inviting recipe that I hope you enjoy as much as I do.

Blend the pulp from a green juice until smooth. I like to use the pulp from my green machine juice (see page 14).
Add an extra-large handful of fresh mint leaves and 1 drop of peppermint 100% pure essential oil. Continue blending until smooth.
Add 1/2 cup of raw walnuts, 1/2 cup raw pecans, 1/2 cup raw hazelnuts, and continue blending.
Add 8 pitted medjool dates with 1/3 cup coconut sugar and continue blending.
Add 1 cup of almond meal to thicken, and blend together till smooth (may need a touch more almond meal depending on how moist you like your slice to be).
The coconut pulp left over from making your own coconut milk (see page 11) also works really well in this recipe as an alternative to almond meal. I sometimes include 1 cup of the coconut milk pulp here as well as the almond meal, or you could add 1/2 a cup of desiccated coconut.
Place mixture in a non-stick square or rectangular baking tray (I still line my tray with baking paper to allow easier removal of the slice from the baking tray).

Icing:
I blend together:
3 ripe avocado
1/2 cup raw cacao powder
8 pitted medjool dates

Blend until thick and smooth, then spread over the top of the mint slice.
Place in freezer for 30 minutes to set.
When ready to serve, take out of the freezer and use the baking paper to carefully pull the slice from the baking tray. Cut into even squares and place on serving plate. Eat chilled, enjoy!
Note: an extra garnish of cacao nibs on top goes down very nicely!

Fig Delight Cream

I make my own ice cream out of many different fruits and spices.

3 fresh figs, frozen
3 frozen bananas
3 frozen medjool dates, pitted
1/2 cup pure organic coconut cream (optional for extra creaminess)

Blend all together till thick, creamy and smooth. Garnish with fresh figs and enjoy!

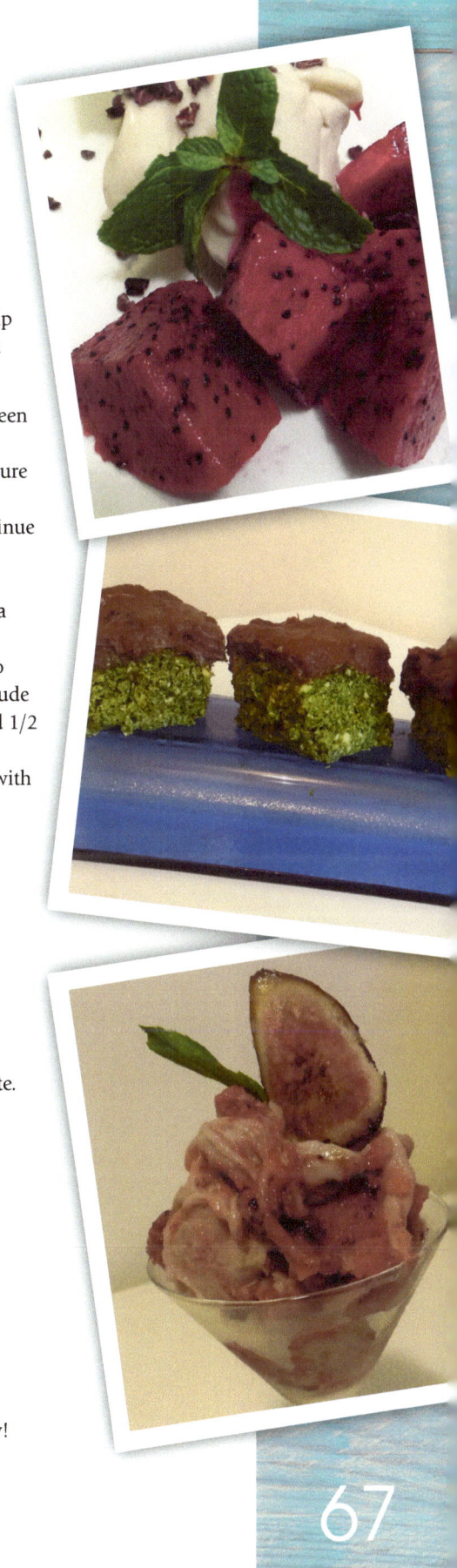

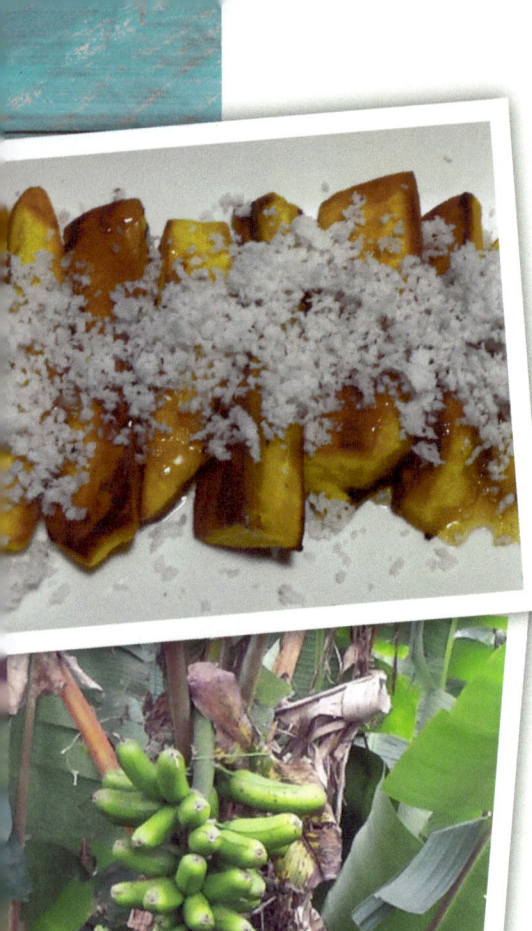
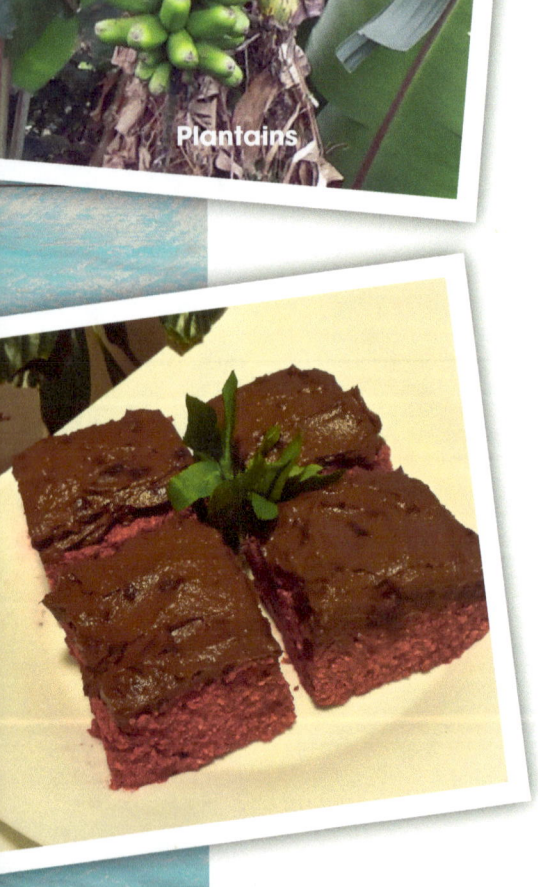

Plantains

Warm Plantain Fingers - my little taste of Fiji

Inspired by my travels in the beautiful islands of Fiji, this simple and tasty dessert is a hearty nourishing comfort treat rich in flavour. I've been eating plantains since I first discovered them on my overseas travels – they are actually a natural super food that many people are unaware of (see page 77 plantain benefits).

3 ripe plantains
1 generous drizzle raw honey
2 cups fresh scraped coconut or coconut milk pulp

Slice plantains in half longways and then in half again until you have several 'fingers', and grill or BBQ on both sides until toasty and golden. Place the cooked plantains on a serving dish, drizzle with raw honey and sprinkle with fresh scraped coconut.
Delicious tastes of paradise melting in your mouth!

Raw Cherry Ripe Slice

This slice tastes so good, even if I do say so myself! It really has that cherry ripe taste and texture, but with a whole lot of wholesome nourishing goodness.

I blend:
2 large fresh red beetroot
2 cups fresh cherries, pitted (when in season)
8 pitted medjool dates
1/3 cup coconut sugar

1 cup raw, cold-pressed organic coconut oil (liquid form)
1 cup raw macadamia
1 cup raw hazelnut
2 cup desiccated coconut, or use the coconut pulp left over from making your own coconut milk (see page 11)

Note: Use more desiccated coconut or coconut milk pulp if needed to thicken up slice mixture.
Place the mix in a non-stick square or rectangular baking tray. I line my tray with baking paper to allow even easier removal of the slice from the tray.

Topping
3 ripe avocado
1/2 cup raw cacao powder
8 pitted medjool dates
1/2 cup cacao nibs
Blend then spread the topping over the cherry slice, making it into delicious cherry ripe slice.
Place in freezer for half an hour to set.

When ready to serve, take out of the freezer and use the baking paper to carefully pull out the slice from the baking tray. Cut into even squares, place on serving plate. Eat chilled and enjoy!

Deconstructed Raw Banoffee Pie

I make my raw deconstructed banoffee pie in three stages then layer them in a tall glass so all the elements can be easily viewed – it tastes just as delicious as it looks. I absolutely love this dessert. Hard to believe it's made from parts of edible plants and fruits isn't it? Yum yum yum!

Base
Blend and mix well together:
1 handful raw almonds
1 handful raw cashews
1 handful raw macadamia nuts
6 pitted medjool dates
1/4 cup purified water

Caramel
Blend and mix together:
8 pitted medjool dates, pre-soaked in water for 15min
1 handful raw cashews
2 tbsp coconut sugar
2 tbsp purified water

Cream
Make banana delight cream (see page 65).
Serve in a tall glass layering the base, the cream and then the caramel.
Decorate with fresh slices of banana, cacao nibs or crushed raw pecan nuts for extra crunch.
Note: this dessert is best enjoyed chilled. Make this dessert just before you are about to serve it so that the 'cream' is eaten at its best chilled texture.

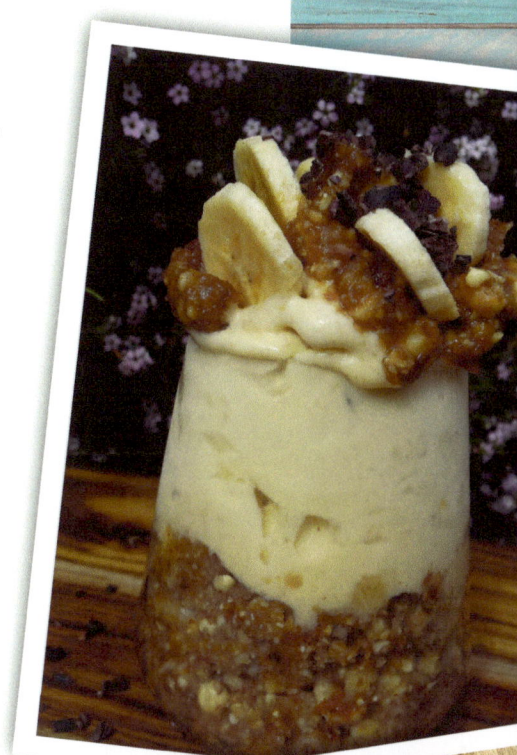

Carambola Star Fruit or Fuji Persimmon and Fresh Fig Chocolate Fondue

This is a great healthy dessert alternative for any dinner party, family gathering, even a kid's birthday. It's healthy and nutritious, but I love how it's a novelty dish and creates excitement. I remember having cheese fondue and chocolate fondue as a child and loved it. This dish is a reminder of my childhood days, but I've created my own style with a super healthy twist that tastes amazing. I use bamboo skewers to pierce and dip the fruit.

For 2 to 3 people I prepare:
3 carambola (or star fruit) or
2 fuji persimmon
3 fresh figs
Cut the fruit into chunks and place on large serving board, then in small serving bowl melt:
1 cup raw, cold-pressed organic coconut oil (1 1/2 cups if in liquid state) and add 3/4 cup raw cacao powder to melted coconut oil, mixing together to create the chocolate dip for the fondue. Then place into small dipping bowls:
1 handful cacao nibs
1 handful raw pistachios, roughly crushed
1 handful raw almonds, roughly crushed

Pierce fruit onto bamboo skewers, dip into the warm chocolate mix then roll over cacao nibs, pistachio pieces, crushed almonds or shredded coconut and enjoy this guilt free fondue experience!

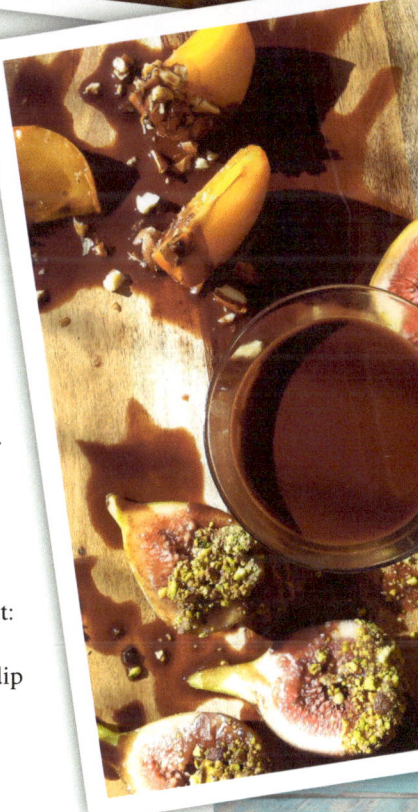

Transformation is not just physical, it's mental. Your mind has to believe first.

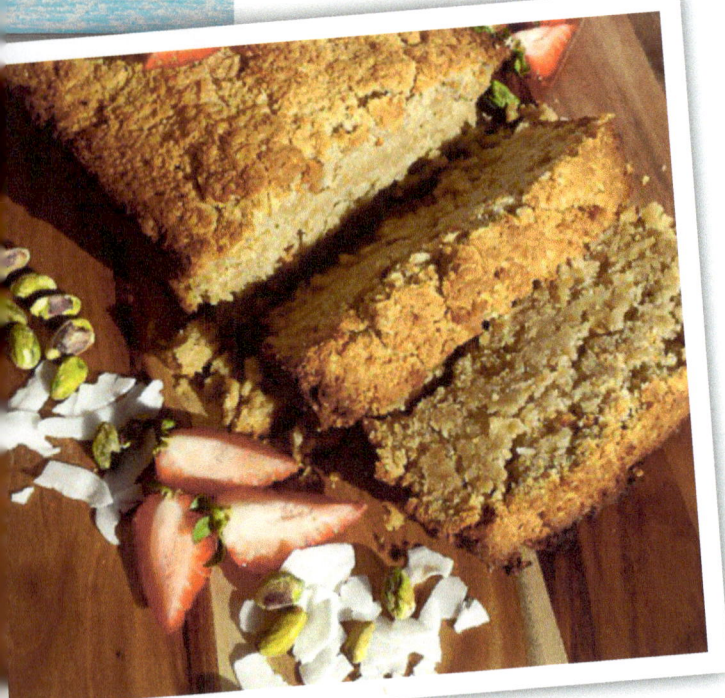

Honey Comb Rhubarb Crumble Loaf

I love the texture and aromas of this loaf. It's dairy free, refined sugar free, there's no flour used, only all natural nourishing ingredients – it's guilt free. This cake just ticks all the right boxes!

1 bunch fresh rhubarb stalks
200g fine desiccated coconut
4 cups organic rolled oats
450g almond meal
4 tbsp raw honey
1 large piece (roughly hand-sized) of raw honeycomb
1 small pinch of pink Himalayan salt
6 heaped tbsp raw, cold-pressed organic coconut oil (or 12 if in liquid state)
1 handful raw pistachios
6 fresh strawberries

Chop rhubarb into pieces and boil it, covering the pieces with just enough water.
Cook till slightly soft and stringy.
In a separate bowl, combine desiccated coconut and almond meal. Add pinch of salt.
Melt coconut oil in a separate bowl.
Add cooked rhubarb, including the cooking water, to the dry ingredients. The water that the rhubarb is cooked in adds great flavour. Stir all together.
Add melted coconut oil and raw honey. Stir through. Add raw honeycomb after breaking it up a bit with a fork. Stir. The raw honeycomb will melt through the mixture while in the oven, so don't worry if it's in small clumps while preparing this mixture
Gradually add rolled oats to thicken and continue to stir.
Line a baking tray with baking paper. When the mixture is thick yet still moist, pour onto the lined tray. Place in oven.
Bake for 1 1/2 – 2 hours at 180 degrees, keeping an eye on the loaf by turning it around occasionally so the sides cook evenly and don't burn. After an hour of cooking, pierce the loaf with a skewer to test how it is cooking on the inside.

This loaf takes a little while to cook, but it's so quick and easy to whip up and put together. While waiting for it to cook, I always go about my housework or other activities, or even throw in a quick home workout – in no time at all the loaf is cooked. When ready, take out of oven and leave to cool for half an hour in the baking tray to maintain the shape of the loaf. Remove from the baking tray using the baking paper. I like to place on wooden serving board and serve with fresh strawberries, coconut flakes and raw pistachios.
Note: This loaf keeps in sealed container in the fridge for up to 10 days, or shelf life up to 5 days

Frosty Fruit Royale

These gorgeous dessert treats are the perfect 'after dinner mint' substitute. The fresh delicious fruit layers make this an attractive and nourishing finish to any main meal. You can use any fruit you like, but the idea is to create inviting colour. I like to make my frosty fruit royale like this...

Using my mini chopper I blend:
1 small banana until creamy and smooth, placing it in the bottom of each of my ice block moulds
1 kiwifruit till smooth, placing that on top of the banana in the moulds
1 small handful strawberries until smooth, placing that on top of the kiwifruit in the moulds
1 hand-sized piece of paw paw or mango until smooth, placing it on top of the blended strawberries in the moulds

Add bamboo sticks gently into the mixture in the moulds and place in freezer for 4 hours or till frozen.
I like to dip the tip of my frosty fruit royales into a mix of 1/4 cup raw cacao powder and 1 tablespoon of raw, cold-pressed organic coconut oil, melted and stirred together.
Finish with a decorative roll in crushed nuts of choice or cacao nibs, desiccated coconut or organic activated plain buckinis.
Place back in the freezer for a few minutes to set the cacao and nuts into place and until ready to eat – best eaten chilled like ice-blocks. Enjoy!

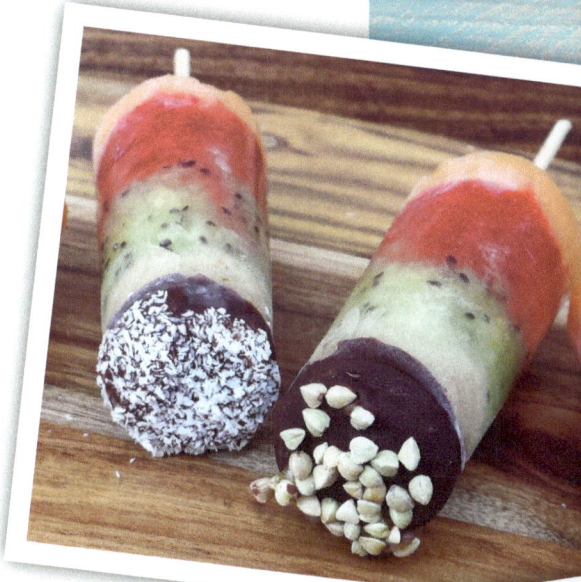

Papaya Bliss balls

The beauty of these succulent papaya bliss balls is how fresh and moist they are. I made these with the abundance of fresh fruit and coconut in Fiji and it sure made a lasting impression. Using freshly scraped coconut just takes these treats to another level.

1 fresh coconut, freshly scraped (you could use 2 cups desiccated coconut as a substitute, mixed with just over 1/2 cup raw, cold-pressed organic coconut oil, or better still use the coconut milk pulp from making coconut milk but to get the best flavour and texture from these delicious Papaya bliss balls freshly scraped coconut is what I use.)
1 medium-sized fresh papaya, seeds removed and flesh mashed (don't throw seeds away, see page 77)
1 handful medjool dates, chopped
1 handful dried figs, chopped
1 cup crushed raw almonds
3/4 cup raw, cold-pressed organic coconut oil (in its liquid state)
1 generous drizzle raw honey to taste
1 sprinkle organic cinnamon

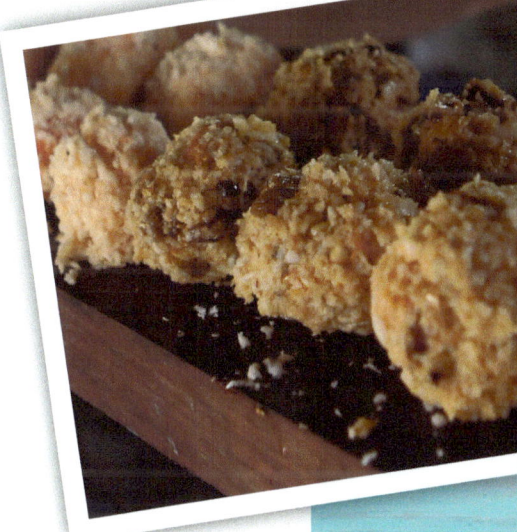

Gently mix all ingredients until well combined, using 3/4 of the freshly scraped coconut.
With clean hands, roll the mix into balls.
Roll the balls over the remaining coconut, place on a serving board and pop in the fridge for 45 minutes or until set.
These are best eaten when freshly-made, but will keep in the fridge in sealed container for up to 5 days.
Note: drizzle a tad more raw honey over the bliss balls on the serving board when ready to serve for an impressive finishing touch.

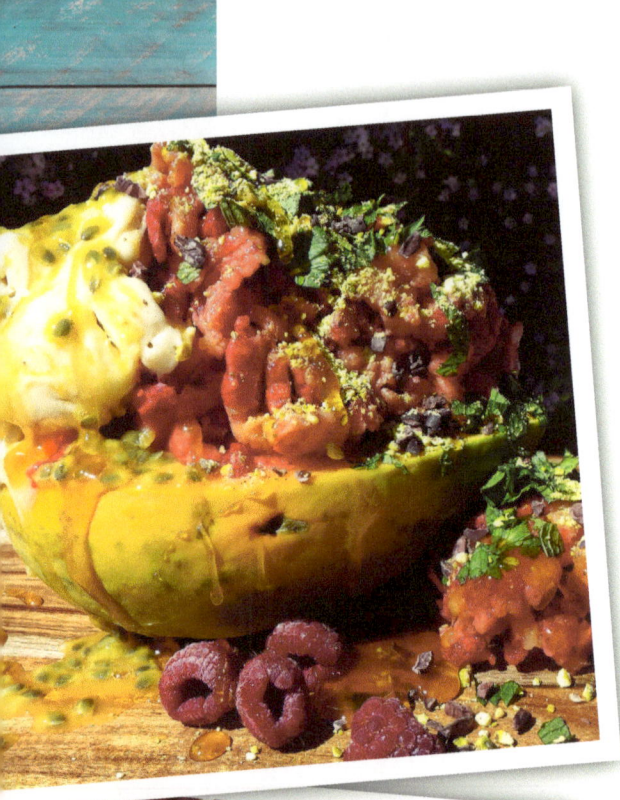

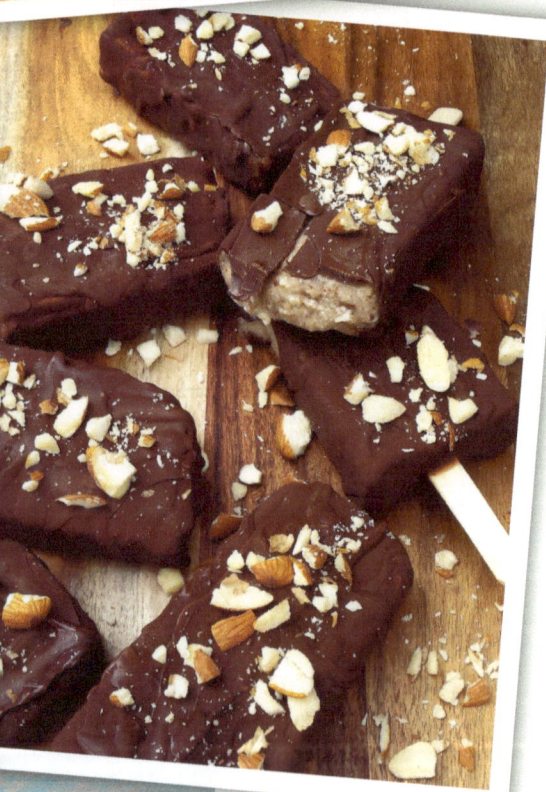

Summer Paw Paw Pleasure Boats

I always have pre-prepared fresh fruits to freeze and have on hand when I need them. This dessert is one that I absolutely must have during those hot, humid summer days – it really hits the spot!

For these Summer Paw Paw Pleasure Boats you will need -
1 half of a fresh paw paw, seeds removed (but don't throw seeds away. See page 77)
1 large handful of frozen paw paw slices
1 handful frozen strawberries
1 handful frozen raspberries
1 batch of banana delight cream (see page 65)
1 passionfruit
1 handful fresh mint, finely chopped
1 drizzle raw honey
1 tsp crushed pistachios
1 tsp cacao nibs

Place the frozen paw paw slices, frozen strawberries and frozen raspberries into blender and blend till thick and smooth.
Slice a fine slither of skin off from the underneath of the remaining fresh paw paw half so that it sits steadily on a serving board acting as the boat.
Scoop frozen blended mix of paw paw, strawberries and raspberries into the fresh paw paw half.
Add scoops of banana delight cream also into the fresh paw paw half.
Drizzle over fresh passionfruit and sprinkle finely chopped fresh mint along with 1 drizzle raw honey, and a sprinkle of crushed pistachios and cacao nibs to finish this dessert off with a delicious mouth-watering tasty crunch.

Chocolate Coated Banana and Cinnamon Pops

So easy to make and they taste so good! These guilt-free chocolate-coated banana and cinnamon 'ice-creams' offer a satisfying and delicious finish to any evening meal.

Make one batch of 'Morning Pow' (see page 22) and pour into moulds.
Place the moulds in the freezer overnight to set.
When ready to serve mix together:
1 heaped tbsp raw cacao powder with 1/2 cup of melted raw, cold-pressed organic coconut oil until well combined.
Take the 'ice-creams' out of the moulds and dip them into the mixture of cacao powder and coconut oil and rest them on a plate. Decorate with crushed almonds.
Place the plate back into the freezer for a further five minutes for the 'chocolate' to set.
Take out of freezer when ready to eat, enjoy!

Raw Coconut Rough Ice cream with Broken Chocolate

That coconut rough chocolate experience when I was a child must have made a lasting impression on me, because even today I remember the taste. This ice cream, delight cream, is my version of all those exciting memories and flavours I remember having as a child. A healthy version of golden coconut rough? Who would have thought! And all from nourishing edible plants.

I simply use:
1/2 cup desiccated coconut
1/2 cup coconut sugar
1/2 cup purified water

Blend all together really well then add:
1 very generous drizzle of coconut syrup
Blend together again until the mixture becomes golden, thick and smooth.
Place blended mixture into a cake tin and put into freezer. Leave in freezer for 3 hours or till well frozen.
I use mini square loose-based cake tins, but really you can use any size cake tin, preferably on the smaller side. After the mixture has frozen, just cut it into blocks. The mini cake tins just make life a little easier and save you from having to slice your own blocks of ice cream.

Just before removing the ice cream from the freezer, I prepare:
1 cup raw cacao powder added to 1 1/2 cups raw, cold-pressed organic coconut oil (melt coconut oil if not already in liquid form)
Stir these together until combined.
Remove frozen mixture from cake tin, slice into blocks if need be, and place blocks onto a serving board. Drizzle the cacao and coconut oil mixture all over the ice cream blocks. I like to coat the blocks this way as it gives this dessert more character.
Place back into the freezer for five minutes to set. The cacao coating should crack as it sets, creating that broken chocolate effect. Take out of the freezer just before eating and decorate with shredded coconut and cacao nibs – enjoy!

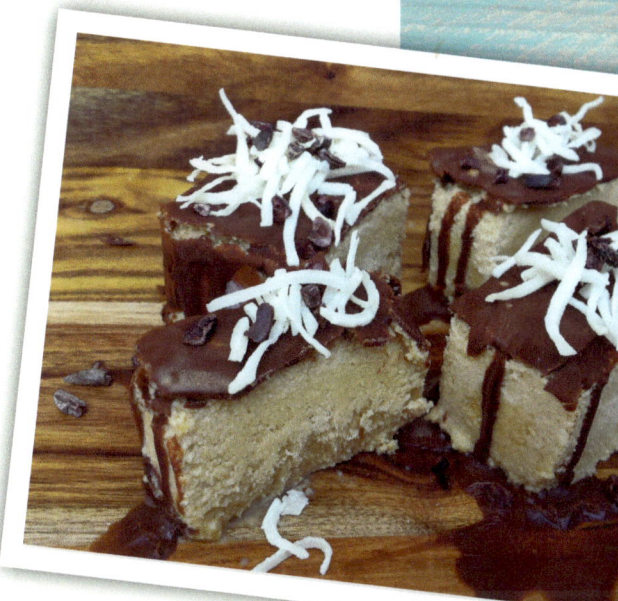

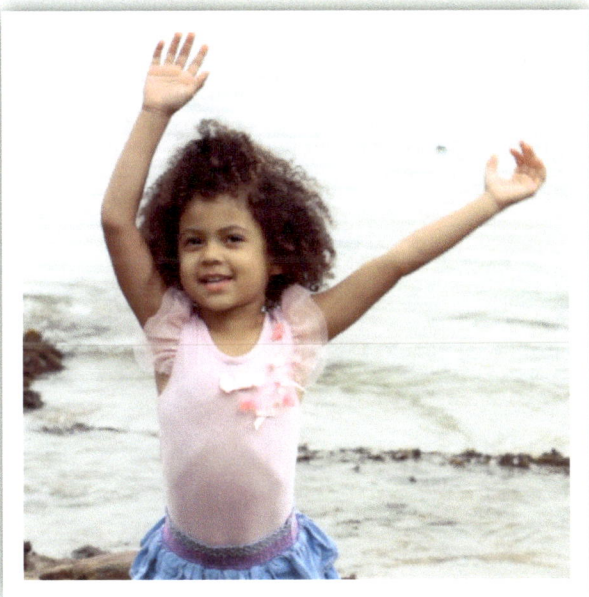

Remember why you started this journey, then remind yourself why you choose to see it through

Adore Teas, Herbs and Useful Uses

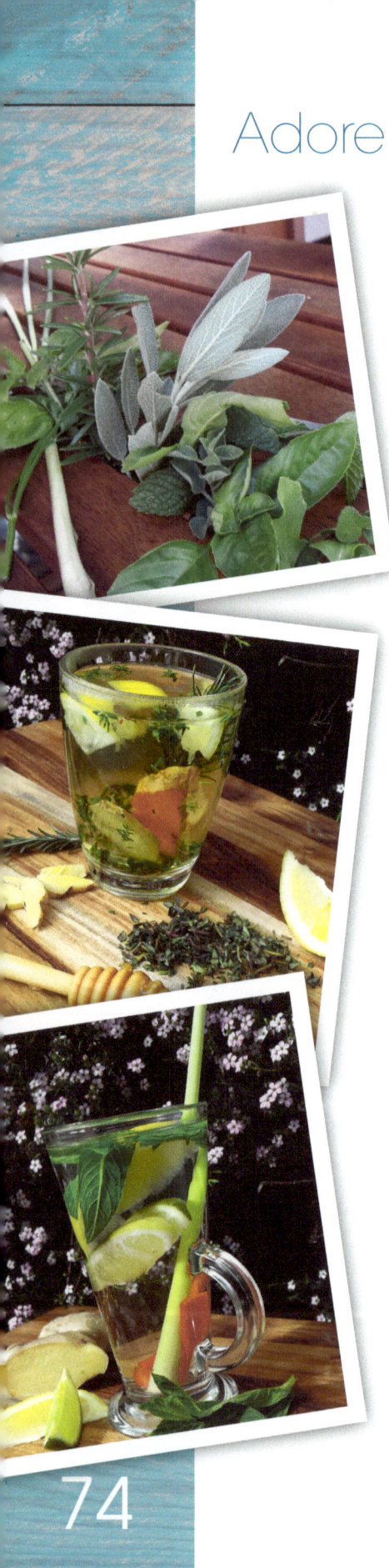

Herbs and spices to have on hand

Turmeric, fresh ginger, cracked black pepper, pink Himalayan salt, organic cinnamon, fresh rosemary, fresh thyme, fresh mint, fresh chilli, fresh lemon grass, cayenne pepper, paprika, cumin, fresh sage, star anise, nutmeg.

Oils and natural dressings to have on hand

Raw apple cider vinegar, fresh lemons and limes, pure organic virgin olive oil, raw cold-pressed organic coconut oil, organic balsamic vinegar, flaxseed oil, a selection of 100% pure essential oils such as peppermint, lavender, orange and lemon.

Natural Cough Remedy Tea

1 thumb-sized piece of fresh ginger, cut into slices
1 thumb-sized piece of fresh turmeric, cut into slices
1 small handful fresh thyme
1 small handful fresh rosemary
1 fresh lemon, squeezed
1 tsp raw organic honey

Place all dry ingredients into a tea cup. Add fresh lemon juice and lemon pulp bits into tea cup. Dangle the teaspoon of honey over tea cup, pouring boiling water over the spoon. The honey will melt off and dissolve into the tea cup ingredients. Fill the cup to the brim with boiling water. Enjoy!
Add a drop of lemon or orange 100% pure essential oil to the cup of tea to assist with further relief
Turmeric is such a powerful spice. The use of turmeric in cooking helps maintain health and fight off disease.

Vietnamese Inspired Sore Throat Cure Tea

The amazing aromas and flavours of the exotic foods in Vietnam that I experienced brought about the inspiration for this delicious tea that soothes and eases the throat so well.

1 thumb-sized piece of fresh ginger, cut into slices
1 fresh lemon, squeezed
1 fresh lime wedge
1 stalk of lemongrass, chopped in half to release the flavour
1 handful fresh mint
1 chopped red chilli, stem removed
1 drizzle of raw honey (optional to sweeten – it really does taste amazing as is)

Place all dry ingredients into tea cup. Add fresh lemon juice and lemon pulp bits into tea cup. Dangle the teaspoon of honey over tea cup, pouring boiling water over the spoon. The honey will melt off and dissolve into the tea. Fill the cup to the brim with boiling water. Enjoy!
*a drop of lemon 100% pure essential oil can also be added

Healthy Heart Tea

Inspired by my travels in the beautiful islands of Fiji

In a tea cup, add boiling water to:
1 clean hibiscus flower
1 lemon tree leaf (bent in half to bring out more flavour)
2 kaffir lime leaves (bent in half to bring out more flavour)
3 fresh lavender flowers
1 wedge of fresh lime

Wait for two to three minutes for the flavours to come alive in the hot water, then sip to your heart's content.
*a drop of lavender 100% pure essential oil can be added to this healthy heart tea

Orange Comfort Tea

This tea was inspired by the freezing cold winter days that I survived during my time in the UK!

Place the following ingredients into a tea cup:
8 cloves
4 star anise
1 organic cinnamon stick
2 or 3 slices of a fresh ripe orange (use the rest of the orange to squeeze as described in the next preparation step)
2 tbsp of fresh orange juice
1 tbsp orange rind
1 tspn roughly grated nutmeg
1 tspn coconut sugar

Cover with boiling water and stir.
Enjoy the absolute inner comfort this warm tea provides. Great on those cold nights in front of an inviting fire, or simply just to warm the body up.
*you can also add two kumquats cut in half if desired along with a drop of orange 100% pure essential oil

Peppermint Tea Naturally – The Stomach Settler

Try this tea when an upset stomach is getting the best of you.
It's really simple to make.

1 handful fresh mint leaves
1 tsp dried peppermint leaves
1 thumb-sized piece of fresh ginger (fresh ginger adds an extra spark to this tea)

Place all ingredients into a tea cup or mug, add boiling water and give a stir. Relax and let the tea work its soothing magic.
*adding a drop of peppermint 100% pure essential oil to this tea is ideal

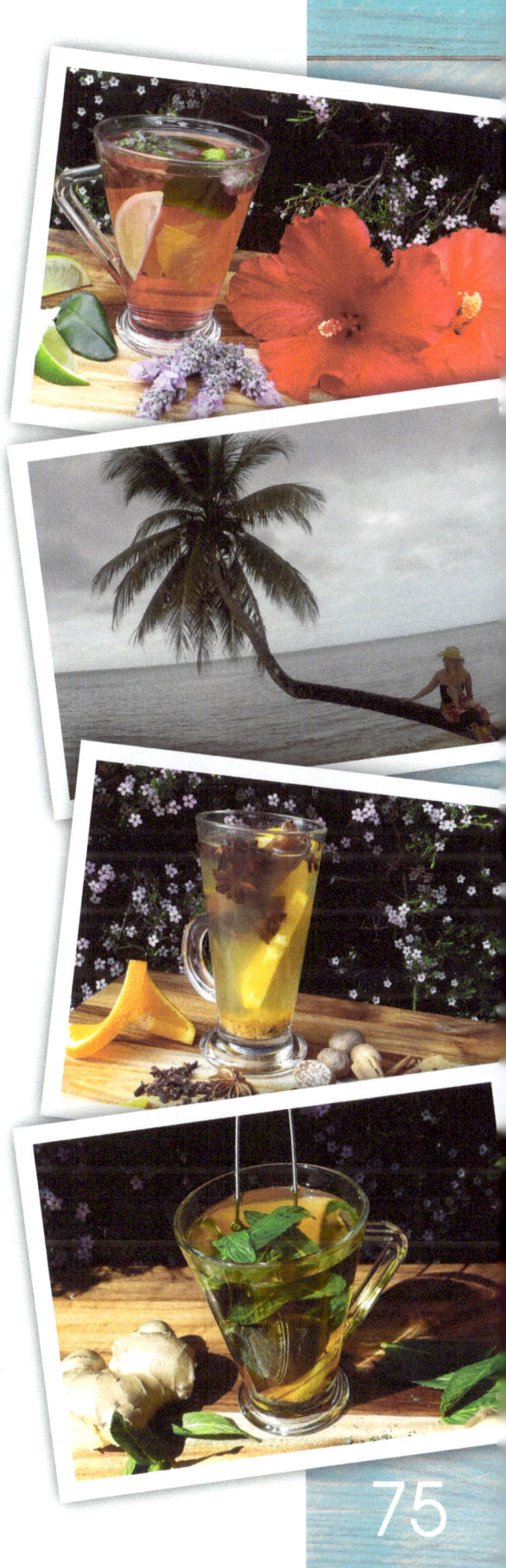

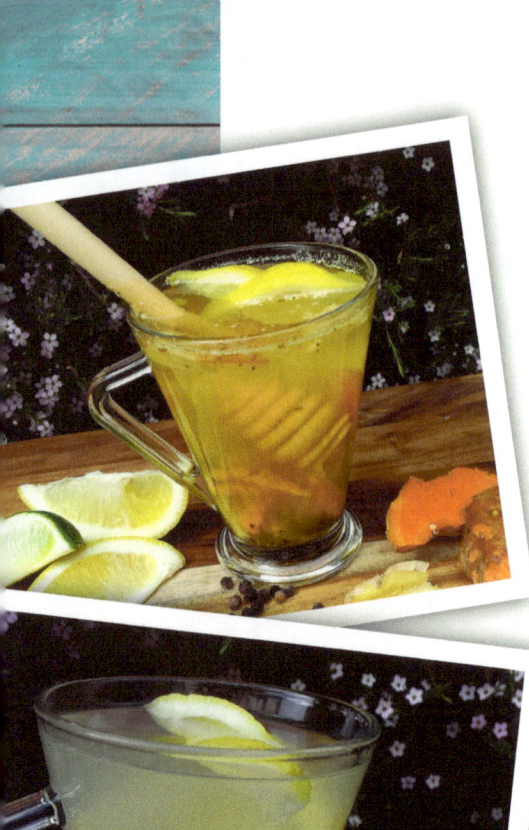

Turmeric Tea
Healing & Health Tea

1 thumb-sized piece of fresh turmeric, chopped
1 thumb-sized piece of fresh ginger, chopped
The juice of 1/2 a lemon
2 fresh lemon slices
1 tsp raw honey
1 sprinkle cracked black pepper

Place all ingredients in tea cup. Dangle the teaspoon of raw honey over the tea cup pouring boiling water over the spoon. The honey will melt off and dissolve into the. Fill to the brim with boiling water, stir and enjoy!

Essential Warm Lemon Water

Drinking this of a morning wakes up the senses and gets the metabolism fired up!

Boil kettle, then as it is cooling slightly prepare:
1 fresh lemon, juiced
Optional: add extra lemon wedges if desired or fresh ginger

Pour the fresh lemon juice into a tea cup, add warm water and lemon wedges, as well as a drop of lemon 100% pure essential oil.
Enjoy first thing in the morning to revitalise your digestive system and get your metabolism pumped up and working.

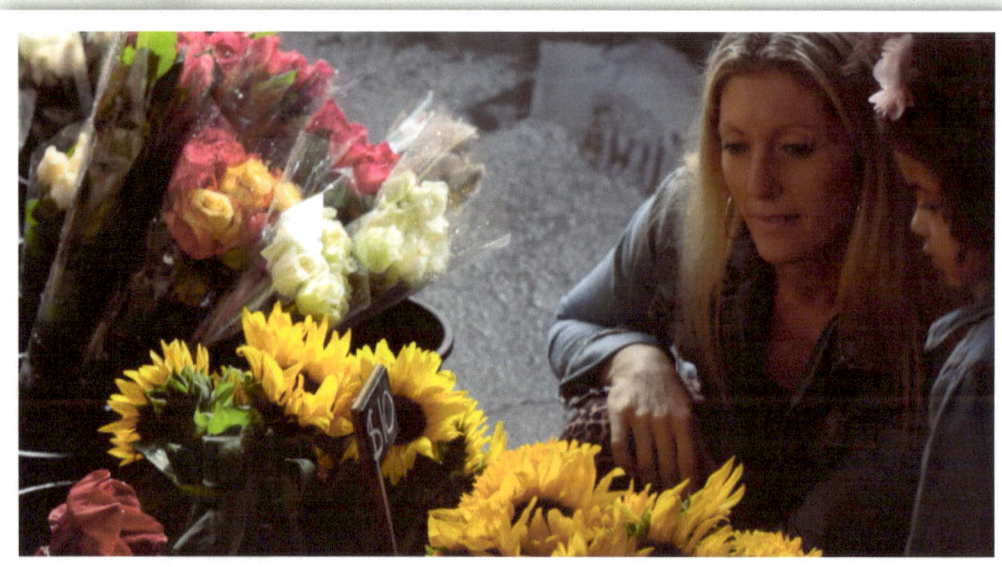

My Love for Herbs and Spices

My love for herbs and spices began with many special times in my childhood. There are several occasions that stand out to me very clearly, where the opportunity was given to experience incredible authentic tastes of many cultural dishes where herbs and spices were at their best. The memory of experiencing these diverse and incredibly unique flavours has stayed with me in my own health, cooking and lifestyle choices.

There is always a natural alternative for everything. These are a few of the many natural herbs, spices, fruits and plants I have found helpful, along with their amazing health benefits.

BLACK PEPPER – helps reduce body fat, a good digestive stimulant
TURMERIC, RED CLOVER – good for cleansing the blood
TUMERIC - helps rid dermatitis, good for cleansing the blood, fights toxins, improves complexion, helps assist in reducing body fat
BAY LEAF – speeds up wound healing, protects the body from bacterial infections, improves heart health, alleviates respiratory issues, can give relief from anxiety
BARLEY - increases faeces bulk
BASIL - effective relief from asthma or bronchitis, the juice of basil leaves can also help bring down high temperatures
FENNEL, DILL – good for increasing breast milk
CARDAMOM – a good digestive stimulant
ROSEMARY – cough reliever, enhances memory and concentration
CORIANDER - a great thirst reliever and skin circulation improver
DATES AND POMEGRANATE – helps relieve fatigue
DRY GINGER, CAYENNE – great digestive agents
MANGO - heart tonic
RAISINS, PRUNES - natural laxatives
LEMON - improves sense of taste
MINT - great reliever of malaise
MUNG BEANS – for revitalising
PLANTAIN – good for getting rid of dermatitis, helps with menstrual relief, helps prevent kidney and bladder problems
PAW PAW / PAPAYA SEEDS – helps rid body of parasites and worms
DRAGON FRUIT – excellent for treating coloured hair. Simply put the juice on your scalp. It keeps the hair follicles open, allowing hair to breathe and maintain its health and smoothness. Dragon fruit combined with cucumber juice and raw honey is a great moisturiser for relief of sunburnt skin.
SUNFLOWER SPROUTS – encourages clearance of the lungs, a natural expectorant for chest congestion and respiratory infections
HIMALAYAN SALT – helps alkalise the body and regulates hydration

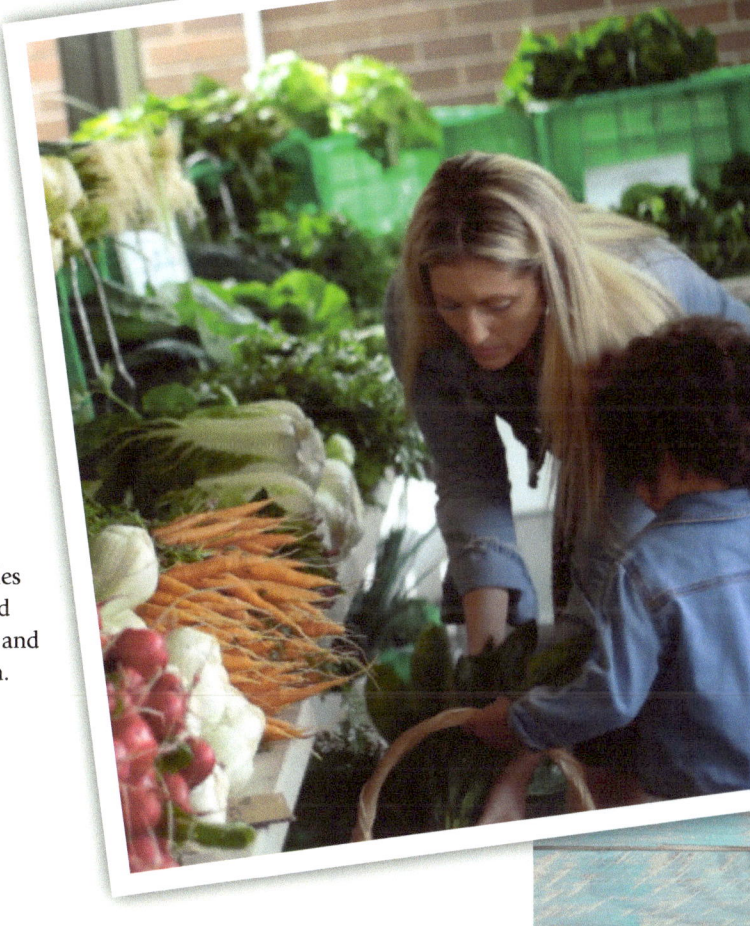

Adore Life

It's easy to forget at times, when the struggle and the pain becomes real, why you started your health and fitness journey. It can be too overwhelming - way too easy to fall into temptation and just throw in the towel. So, I often keep these tips close by to remind myself of the journey I set out on. I set out to see it through to the end - knowing all the while that the obstacles that arise along the way can only have power over me if I allow them to.

When you realise you have the strength to do anything you put your mind to, miracles happen....

- understand that circumstance is temporary
- see situations as opportunities, always looking for the best in them
- let go of anger, jealousy, bitterness, resentment – you become what you hold on to
- look for ways to give, not to get
- avoid judging
- always try your absolute best
- know and embrace your worth
- stay humble and real, fake is always obvious
- be open to change
- find the positive in everything
- keep things simple, don't over-complicate, don't take on too much at once, pace yourself, prioritise

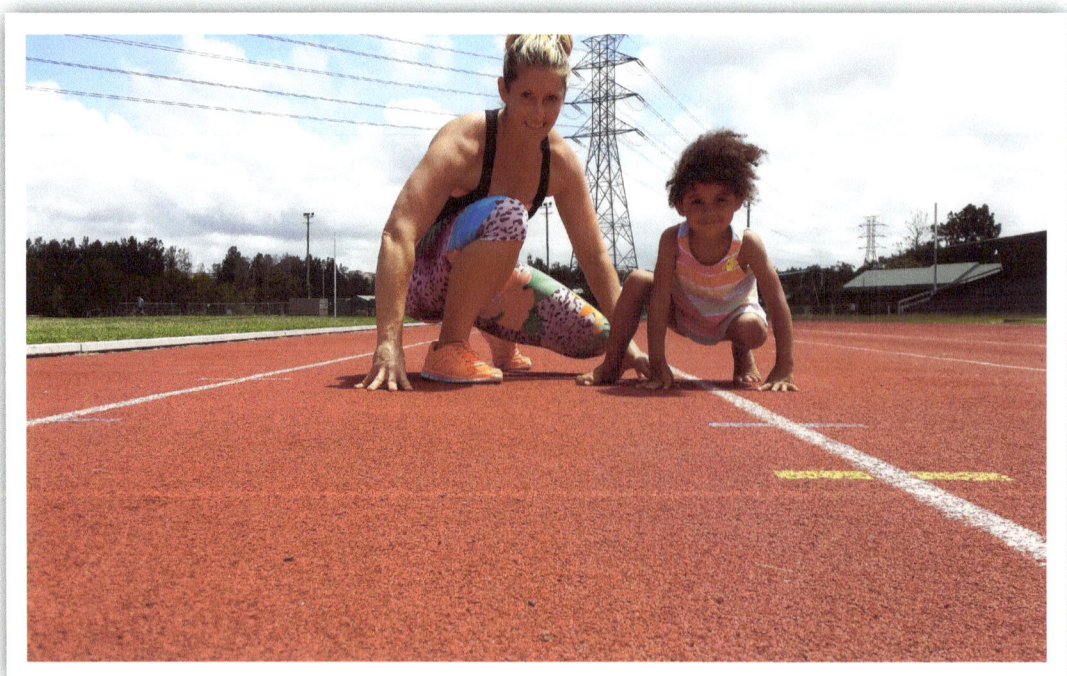

Adore Health... a healthy life starts with healthy thoughts

I spend at least half an hour daily doing something that I love.

I make sure I stay H20 hydrated – it's a great way to ensure your body is working for you, not against you. Staying H20 HYDRATED is super important for fat loss, wellbeing and brain function. I make sure I drink 2.5 litres of purified water daily as a minimum. At least 30 minutes before each meal time or snack I drink a good 1/2 litre of purified water. Not only does it help to keep you fuller for longer, but water flushes out toxins and cleanses the body. Without drinking a good amount of water daily your system simply wont function at its best.

I eat dark leafy greens daily. You can never have enough of the nourishing goodness that assists the whole body in so many ways. I eat as much fresh salad as I can each day (anything fresh and nutritious, straight from nature in its purest and natural state – dark leafy greens and fresh herbs etc.).

I switch off all electronics for a good hour every day. I make time daily to get outdoors, exercise and just breathe fresh air. Enjoying 15 minutes of sun daily for maintaining vitamin D levels just makes me feel amazing! Smiling and laughing is wonderful medicine.

I try to eat every two to three hours with smaller portions - eating until satisfied, never bloated. I listen to my body and what it tells me and when to eat. I'm never afraid of eating fruit – it is nature's natural nourishing goodness gifted to us! The benefits of eating fruit far outweigh the stigma surrounded by eating 'too much' fruit.

Go after your dreams and goals, no matter how hard it may seem, and never give up. Find great inspiration, along with the realisation that we ALL have the potential and ability to better ourselves no matter the obstacle, no matter the impossibilities. Defy your impossible! Adore your lifestyle!

Adore Fitness

Being strong is not just about the weight you can lift or how much you can endure, being strong is a constant positive frame of mind no matter what is going on around you. That alone is strength. Being strong always starts from within.

Practice makes perfect.
Results come from consistency.
Goals are reached through trials, overcoming hurdles and continuously getting up when you've been knocked down! There is no magic quick fix.
I was told at the beginning of my journey back to fitness to consider surgery on my lower stomach.
I struggled, especially at the start, with wondering how I would ever get a flat stomach again after the birth of my daughter.
I have never been one to resort to surgery as an 'option out' of hard work.
So, I put my head down and I worked HARD!
I began with planks, sit-ups, scissor kick exercises, Russian twists... you name it!
I also incorporated HIIT (High Intensity Interval Training).
Sweating is also one of the best ways to drop body fat.
At first I thought nothing was changing, but within 12 short weeks I noticed big changes, and even further down the track, my results have come because of consistency.

Never stop trying!

Some excellent BODY WEIGHT EXERCISES THAT I live by

Easy at home or anywhere exercises

- Fast sprints and short bursts of speed, uphill sprints, on the spot running with high knees, running up sand hills, running up a steep staircase or anywhere with lots of stairs to work the legs
- Deep lunges
- Jumping up stairs and squats going up stairs work wonders for the glutes
- Fast-paced power walks for 45min or more
- On the spot jumping squats - a powerful glute and thigh exercise.
- Burpees are an awesome whole body workout
- Dips and planks for arm toning and firming the stomach area
- Calf raises for tone to the back of legs
- Push-ups and glute raises are fabulous for firming and toning
- Skipping is a great way to burn fat and get fit

I love hanging leg raises! I started doing these daily. Finding a bar to hang from, I started with bringing my knees up as close to my chest as I could. As my strength progressed I started to bring straight legs up as close to my chest as possible. I found hanging leg raises a serious strength builder for that lower abdominal area that is often tricky to tone.

Outdoor workouts are always a fun option, especially when you have young ones. I enjoy getting my training done outdoors for many reasons. The fresh air and space for the youngsters to run about is definitely a bonus at the same time. My daughter often joins in. She loves to be part of the action, and it's always great for kids to see their parents being healthy and active. It betters their chances of taking the healthy and active options in life.

Getting outdoors for a workout regularly with my daughter has proven to be a fabulous bonding time too. It's very satisfying to watch her learn the importance of keeping fit.

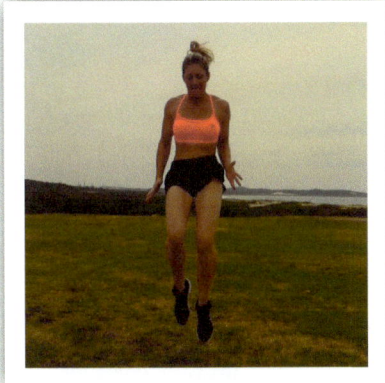 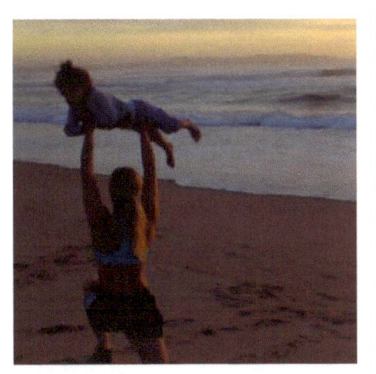 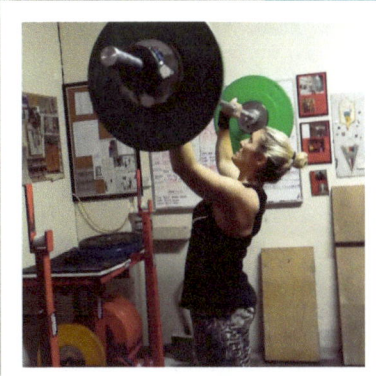

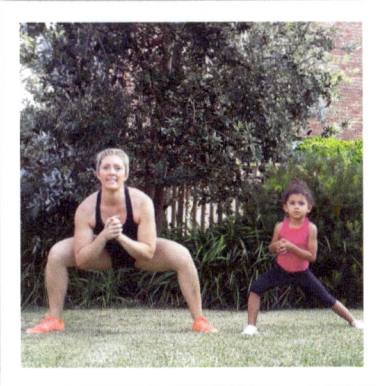 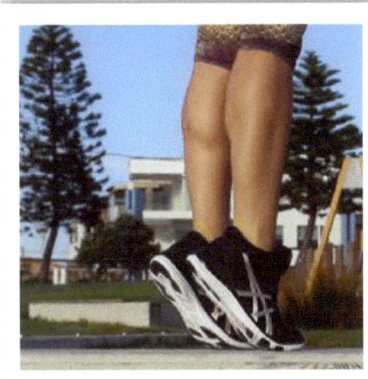 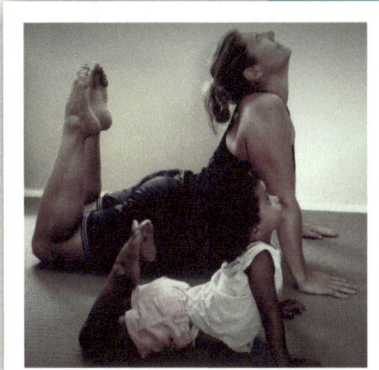

You may not be comfortable going to a gym to workout, or even be able to get to an exercise group. Maybe you don't know where to start with your fitness journey.

For me, I began with my baby, just the two of us. The bonding time is like nothing else and it's such a positive reward for both of us. I know exercising with my daughter has brought better health and quality of life to us both.

Olympic weight lifting came into my life at the perfect time. Having something to challenge me further on my health and fitness journey helped me grow and excel beyond my expectations. Hey, if it isn't taking you out of your comfort zone you can't really expect change! Olympic weight lifting in particular has opened exciting doors to positive challenges and new goals that continue to have positive ripple effects in all areas of my life. It has taught me stronger mental discipline and continues to strengthen my body on a whole new level.

Regular exercise and training, with the inclusion of lifting weights to suit the level of fitness you are at, is so beneficial for the mind and overall health, and the best part is your body will still be burning fat for up to 38 hours after a lifting session.

Go further than where your mind is telling you, the body is capable of so much.

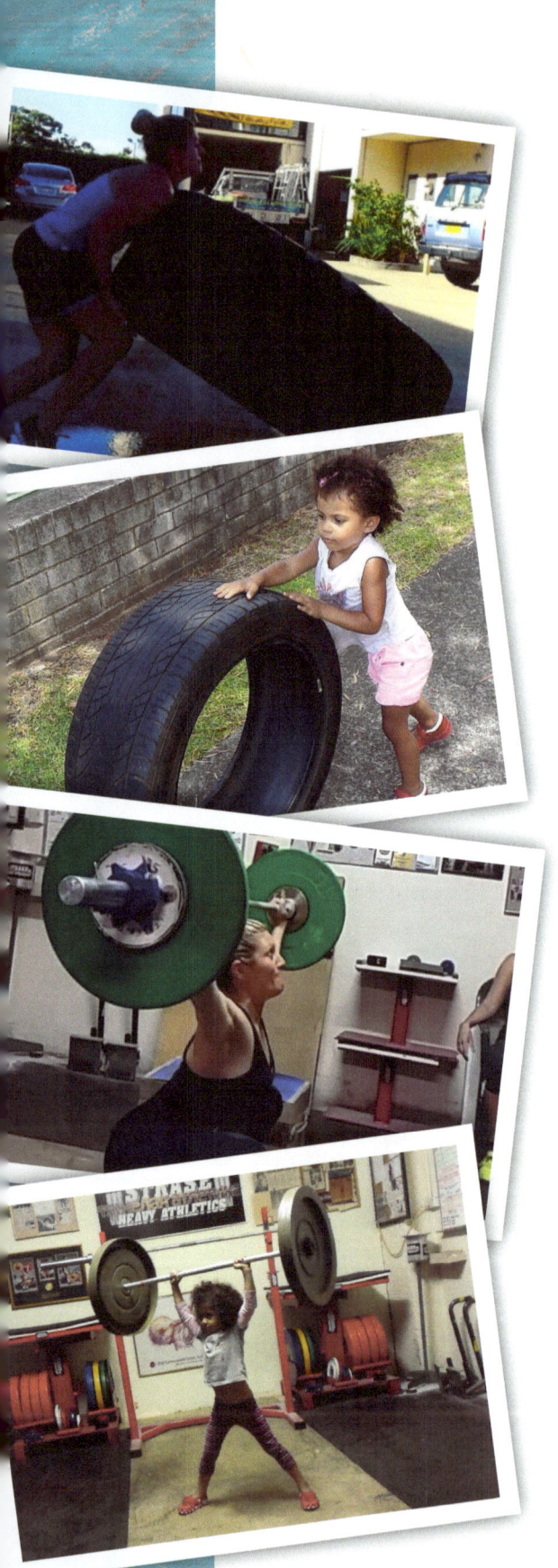

What my typical day looks like – a guide to daily healthy eating and lifestyle

Healthy nourishing food is something I never take for granted, especially when it's available in such abundance and variety. Where there is a plethora of choice, I see it as a responsibility to choose the foods that will heal, repair, restore, create balance and maintain health.

Choosing foods that harm, will do just that – harm!

Every BODY is at a different stage, with different needs and requirements. No one body is the same. What works for one may not always work for another, and it may take time and patience to discover which foods and exercise your body responds best to. What I have discovered over the years, and keep coming back to, is simple – going back to basics is the key.

Whole foods, organic foods, eating foods that grow from the ground, straight from nature, from trees, food in its natural purest state – it's not rocket science.

If we all ate and drank a whole lot more of what nature provided and stopped eating factory produced food, I'm sure there would be a lot less suffering from diet-related illnesses and disease, wouldn't you agree?

Health is something never to take for granted.

Each time you put something in your mouth, you are choosing what you become.

I believe every body has the ability to become its absolute healthiest, because every body has the gift of will power and determination. How will you use yours?

There is always a natural alternative. I believe that all things can be reversed. If there is a health issue or a healing issue, then there is a natural way to reverse the condition that has been growing over time unnoticed.

Reactions, symptoms, cravings – they are all ways your body is trying to let you know it needs something specific or is deficient in something. Take time to listen to what your body is telling you.

I appreciate that everyone is at a different stage of their journey, and the fear of giving up or going without certain foods, or changing lifestyles can be a scary thought. But I know once you decide to make a lifestyle of health your priority, you'll begin to see things in a brand new light. Best of all, you'll start to reap unimaginable benefits both physically and mentally. Besides, who wants to be feeling sluggish and tired and even depressed all the time? Have you ever stopped to think, I mean really think, about the food and drink you are putting into your body? It really is true, what you eat and drink will either heal you or harm you.

This has been said many a time and it is absolute truth – food really is medicine.

Here is what a typical day for me looks like, keeping in mind that I chop and change from time to time to add variety. I use the many recipe options included here in my book.

Morning:
When I wake up of a morning the first thing I do is drink:
1/2 litre of purified water
to flush out toxins and fire up my metabolism, then:
1 cup warm freshly-squeezed lemon water
to help kick start my digestion process for the day, cleanse and boost my immune system, but also because I love my liver and any extra help I can give it I will!

I may do a workout here, or a 15 minute HIIT session, depending on my day and training program at the time.

Then I drink 1 glass of my green juice (see page 14) I want to make sure I'm getting the best energetic and health jumpstart to my day. Green juice sure helps to do that! It's easy to digest so I drink it in the morning on a relatively empty stomach so the nutrients can absorb quickly into my system.

Then I enjoy a delicious Morning Pow (see page 22). This is my protein sustenance hit that keeps me fuller for longer and totally satisfied.

I consume these drinks with at least a 15 minute gap between each, but I aim for at least a 30 minute gap between the green juice and the Morning Pow because I want to get the best energy boost and as many nutrients as possible into my system.

Even if I am rushing out the front door and 'on the run' of a morning, I have each one prepared in separate bottles to drink as my morning goes along. On mornings when time isn't an issue, I love to whip up my smashed avocado and jacket kumara (see page 25) or a delicious omelette (see page 18).

Mid Morning:
Yes, that's right, I drink another 1/2 litre of purified water and wait half an hour before I eat a piece of fruit for my morning snack – usually pineapple, watermelon, orange or pear with some almonds or macadamias and often a handful of mixed seeds such as pumpkin seeds, chia seeds, flaxseeds, sunflower seeds, with some goji berries, or inca berries. Or I dig into one of my many inviting snack recipes (see snacks page 52).

I squeeze in a short workout here of either sprints, hill runs, or even a 45 minute gym session if I'm not heading to training that night. Even a good power walk to get the blood pumping is so beneficial for the whole system. I just make sure I'm getting a sturdy form of exercise in wherever possible.

Midday
Hydrate, hydrate, hydrate – I drink another 1/2 litre of purified water 30 minutes before my midday meal.
I love to eat one of my many main meal creations (see page 26) for my midday sustenance.
I eat well throughout the morning and at midday to keep my energy levels up and take on the fuel that will carry me right to the end of the day. I want my body working for me, not against me.

This lifestyle of health is about nourishing your body and soul, with food playing a huge role in that lifestyle of wellness. It's exhilarating to eat foods that give your body the best chance to live LIFE. It's certainly not about a diet by any means. It's actually a gift we have all been given, the gift that we are alive, the gift of life, so why wouldn't you want to use it the best you can in all areas and look after such a precious gift? Our bodies thrive on nutritious foods and exercise. Our bodies actually thank us for it. Doesn't that speak volumes?

Midday meals for me can be anything from my Pizza of Health (see page 35) to my avocado rice (see page 27) or my coconut pumpkin soup (see page 36), always keeping in mind balance. For instance, if I've eaten sweet potato for breakfast, I won't eat it again for lunch.

Mid Afternoon:
Again I drink another 1/2 litre of purified water half an hour before I eat.
I usually indulge in one of my delicious raw dark choc fruit and nut protein balls (see page 54) or my energy balls (see page 52), or even my apple peanut stack (see page 53), but with so many snack options the choice is plentiful. I might also have a fresh cold pressed juice or smoothie here too (see page 13).

Evening:
I drink another 1/2 litre of purified water. It's so great for flushing out toxins and helping my body function as it should.
I often squeeze in my biggest training session before my evening meal. I work out 4-5 times a week, mostly weight-lifting and sprinting.
I can't wait for my salad or my evening meal because I know it will assist my body with repair and restoration while I'm sleeping. My aim is to give my body the best fuel it needs in order to give it the best rest possible. If I eat a heavy meal at night I often go

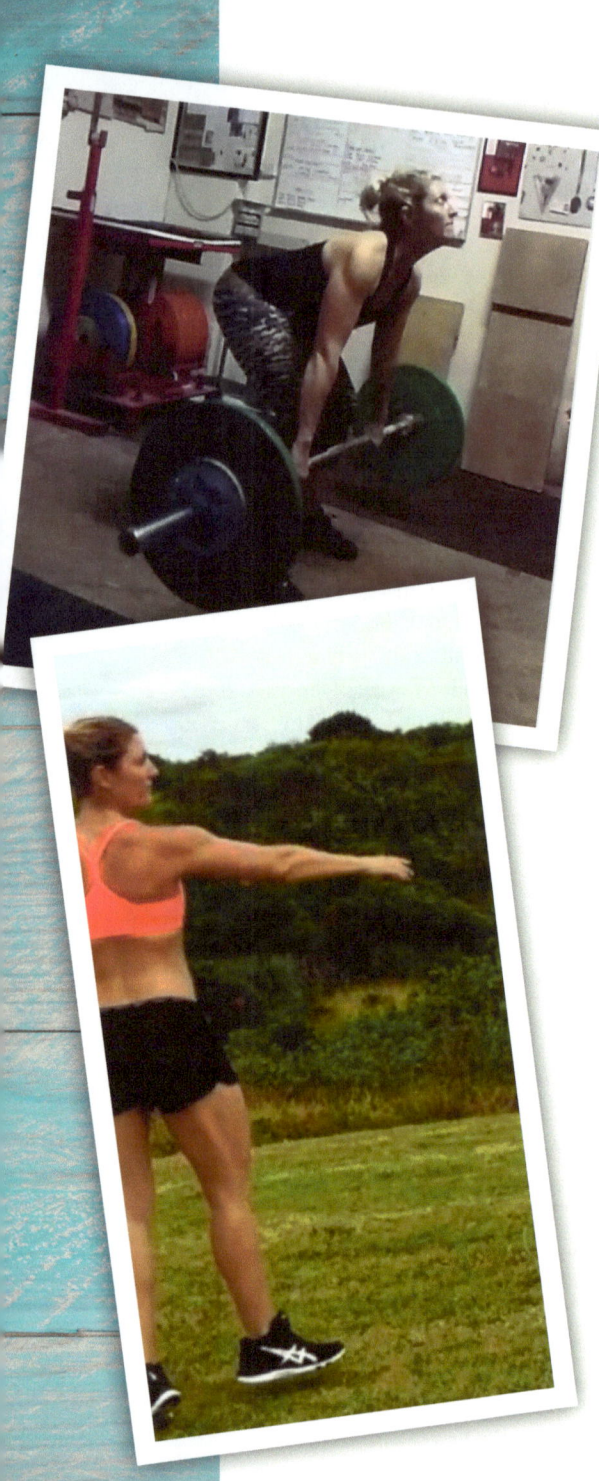

to bed feeling sluggish and bloated, and the night's sleep is spent with my body fighting the effects of that – rather than resting and repairing itself for the next day. This is another reason that I eat my biggest and heaviest meal of the day in the morning or by midday. Ever woken up feeling exhausted? Feeling like you just need to go straight back to sleep again to get over the total lack of energy? A lot of that has to do with the last meal eaten for the day.

I get so excited when I wake up feeling light, refreshed and energised, purely from making a conscious choice to eat well the night before. Food really is medicine, and this is yet another example of how food can heal you or harm you, repair you or deflate you.

My morning and midday meals are a big part of my fuel source to keep me going for the whole day. Eating heavily at night, then sleeping, is like eating the fuel needed before a sports game or a weight-lifting session. If you go to sleep on it, you won't have the chance to burn it off. Repeating this pattern of heavy eating at night before sleep opens the door to weight gain and numerous health issues. Eating right ,especially at night, assists with fat loss and health in more ways than we may be aware. So I think light and satisfying, tasty and content when it comes to fueling my body at night, preparing it to be in the best health it possibly can be for the next day.

My evening meal will consist of anything from my Crispy Tofu and Chilli Stir Fry (see page 28) to my green sprout & lime salad (see page 40)

Bedtime – I drink 1/2 litre of purified water half an hour before I go to bed.

Being healthy and exercising is not about being perfect and trying to get it all right, it's about just starting and then being consistent. Choosing each day to take healthier steps. Deciding daily to continue on the path you've chosen, even when no one else is with you. That's character, that's uniqueness, that's how you bring on change and greatness. That's being an individual and staying true to you. Before long it becomes habit and then you find it is a lifestyle you can't live without.

If you really want something you will do whatever it takes to get it, and it's the same with getting fit and healthy – there are no short cuts. Remember, we are given 24 hours in every day. What will you do with your gift of 24 hours?

It's your journey no one elses.
Only you can defy YOUR impossible...

Endorsements

The Health Train Fiji, Robert and Ginika Fotofili

The most delightful quality about Cat of Ado*raw*ble Treats is that she does not know just how gifted she is. Her mouth-watering recipes are not only a feast for the eyes, but healthy and packed with nutrition. They are a lifeline in these times when even well-fed people are malnourished. Cat is always ready to share her expertise and talents with such passion and humility. She has a generous and caring spirit, which is beautifully illustrated in the detail she pours into her culinary masterpieces. At The Health Train Fiji, we are privileged to call Cat our friend, and we are grateful for the support she has given us, in our joint quest to promote nutritional health as a lifestyle. It is our honour and sincere pleasure to endorse "Adore your lifestyle."

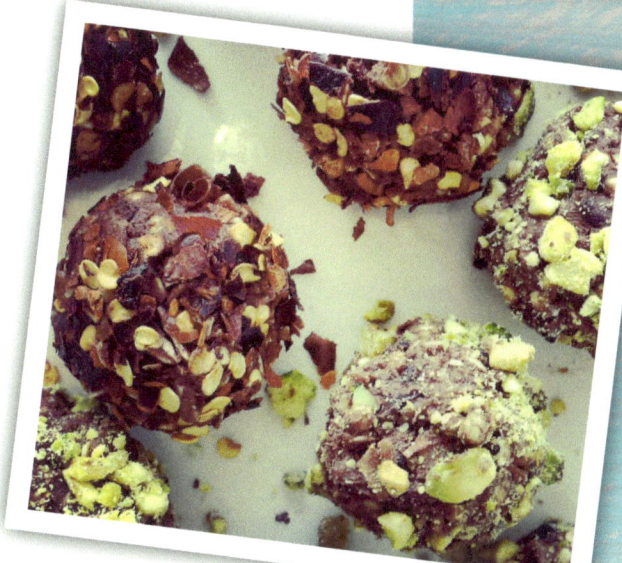

Cecily Paterson, Award winning author of 'Love, Tears & Autism' and 'Invisible'

As one of the many, many people in the world who look somewhat despairingly at their widening waistbands, it sometimes seems impossible that I could ever do anything about my size, let alone do the work I'd need to do to get healthier.

'Those fit people out there must be different from me,' I think. 'They must just have good genes. Or have super willpower. Or something.'

And then I see what Cat has done with her life and her body and this book of nutritious, gorgeous recipes that look like deliciousness on a plate and have lists of beautiful fresh ingredients that go into them – and it's inspiring.

Cat's normal, just like me. She's had a baby belly, just like me. She's trying to make a living, just like me. And yet she's made fitness, weight loss, and glorious, healthy food happen in her life. Cat has embraced new ways to eat and live and work out, and enjoy her life. She's also embraced ethical, nutritious and delicious ways to cook and eat. Quite honestly, she makes the whole thing look less like a diet and much more like a way of life that's fun, honest and yummy at the same time.

I'm impressed with these recipes and tips and I'll be trying them out at home and making changes to the way we eat as a family. I'll also be using her ideas to move more, build my muscle and keep fit and healthy, for the benefit of myself and my kids.

If she can do it, I can do it. And you can too.

N'diaye Talla, Personal Trainer and Nutrition Advisor, London, United Kingdom

Cat is a fantastic person, first of all, but the reason I hold her in high regard is that she is also a great health and lifestyle coach. She has great knowledge about both nutrition and training, but the most important thing for me is the fact that Cat has what I call the 'under the bar' experience. Cat has been at both ends of the spectrum, from a very fit dancer all the way to a post-pregnancy mum. Cat has had to overcome huge obstacles and is now back at her fitness best, proving dedication to a lifestyle of health. Her numerous delicious recipes are absolutely motivating for a lifestyle of health. I know she can inspire you as much as she has inspired me, and help you successfully achieve your goals. Make sure you look out for Cat. She's the inspiration you need for your journey.

Kelly Walker, Nutritional Therapist, Health Hygienist, Natural Health Advisor, Personal Trainer and Former Miss Australia in the International Federation of Body Building

I've tasted lots of Cat's food! Its nutritious, it's delicious, it's convenient and it's really, really tasty. In fact, it has definitely inspired me to start cooking more wholesome foods myself. Cat's original recipes are everything I love about food and eating for a healthy body, mind and lifestyle.

Cat's dedication to her fitness journey and transforming herself has actually inspired me to re-ignite my own fitness journey. I was diagnosed with chronic Lyme Disease which is a life-threatening illness. I had decided to completely stop all my training and was only keeping up with a little bit of nutrition here and there, even though my qualifications told me differently. Again I was inspired by Cat and I began to follow her. Now I'm back into weight training and have lost 8kg. My fitness levels are improving all the time, I'm back to running, I'm doing my cardio again and I'm just feeling a whole lot better overall. I don't think that I would be where I am now if I hadn't been inspired by Cat's journey .

As a therapist myself in nutrition and health, I give credit to Cat on her accomplishments in compiling this book. She is sharing healthy recipes and lifestyle tips that come from her first-hand experiences and knowledge.

Holly Bradley, Wellness Professional specialising in Movement Therapy

I first had the good fortune of meeting Cat not long after the birth of her daughter. Cat was in shock. She had changed dramatically during her pregnancy and was in a place where she knew that she had to make changes to live the lifestyle of health that she wanted. I credit Cat's outstanding results, achieved in a very short amount of time, totally to her willingness to work incredibly hard re-educating herself. She has just kept moving forward; she's amazing! Over the last few years Cat has studied nutrition diligently and her recipes are testament to that. I'm delighted that Cat has finally decided to put her delicious meals into book form, encouraging others to adore a lifestyle of health as she does. Cat has worked incredibly hard with her training, going to astounding places. When you work with her she will back you 1,000 percent. Cat is truly unique because she has that real life experience. She is a very motivated, incredible woman, doing great things in the world and I highly recommend her to everyone I know. I commend her outstanding progress and how she just keeps facing every challenge with such an inspiring, positive attitude.

Belinda Latta – Mum of four, Massage therapist, Independent Younique Presenter and lover of raw organic foods and cruelty-free products.

My personal quest for health and wellness has led me on a minefield journey seeking out 'what is actually healthy' – not just for me, but for my whole family.

Cat has cleverly melded her philosophy of eating predominantly plant-based, raw foods with her talent for executing the most exquisite flavours and combined this with amazing textures, resulting in gorgeous simple recipes suitable for every member of my family, even the littlest ones!

Cat is literally able to breathe a culture into her delicious food and Ado*raw*ble treats. My kids loving every mouthful of these recipes is testament to them tasting every bit as good as they look!

What I love most about Cat's recipes is how her inspiration is drawn from what is left in the fridge, fresh and in season. She keeps things really quick and simple as well as delicious, which is always a plus for a busy mum of four like me.

Trying some of Cat's amazing recipes has literally changed the way I see other raw organic food now.

Cat really has worked everything out to a fine art and presented it in such an easy to use way for every family.

Madonna Hughes, Director, Hypoxi Bodyzone 2007-2012

I've been handing out Cat's recipes to clients at our fitness studio since 2011, I was so impressed with her work and results. Clearly, Cat can cook, and she knows how to eat to get the best of health.

Cat first came to our fitness studio, Hypoxi Body Zone on the Gold Coast, as an embarrassed, disheartened and frustrated lady, after being unable to lose the weight gained from the difficult time during her pregnancy. Less than four months later she walked out, confident, strong and proud, and nearly 30kg lighter! By far our biggest success story, Cat's unbelievable transformation was attested purely to her own determination and commitment to her training and perhaps more importantly – her own healthy eating plan. Initially we gave her some basic nutrition advice which she took further, developing a pure, clean eating plan, perfect for her lifestyle. Each of her meals being packed with the daily essential minerals and vitamins. Cat was such an inspiration to everyone. In the end she was offering other clients advice on nutrition. She was more than happy to hand out her delicious nutritious recipes, which they could not get enough of! She took the hard work out of cooking by providing easy to follow recipes that our clients knew would allow them to eat healthily without 'dieting'.

In the years that followed, Cat has been passionate about healthy wholesome eating, with an insatiable desire to continually develop her knowledge of nutritious food and share it with others. Sparking the idea to put all this knowledge together and create a book filled with delicious, nutritious recipes – one that can inspire anyone to prepare and create healthy, easy meals for themselves and their families. This book is jam-packed with meal ideas that will blow you away, not only because each and every recipe is scientifically good for you, but because each one is also absolutely delicious and full of flavour. With breakfast, lunch, dinner and snacks all covered you will never go hungry again – and never feel guilty either!

The only time you should look back is to see how far you've come.

Special Mention

I source my nourishing healthy ingredients and my food creation inspiration from many places. Organic and farm fresh produce, herbs and spices, oils and whole foods, as well as my training and fitness motivation, have come from these wonderful places and people:

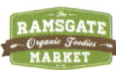 The Ramsgate Organic Foodies Market

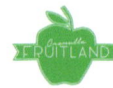 Cronulla Fruitland

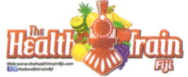 The HEALTH TRAIN Fiji

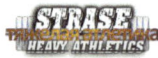 Strase Heavy Athletics

 Oakville Farm Fresh Harvest

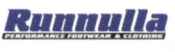 Runnulla

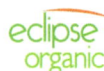 Eclipse Organics

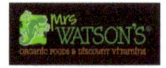 Mrs Watsons

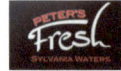 Sariwa Fresh Foods at Ramsgate Organic Foodies Market

Peters Fresh Sylvania Waters

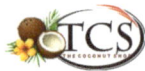 The Coconut Shop

There are also some caring businesses that provide pure, natural organic body creams, natural soaps, oils and other essentials for the body that I just love!

 Sonya Driver – Eco Tan

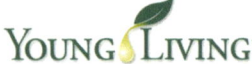 Frank and Anna Kardos – Young Living Essential Oils

TAMANU OIL Nathan at Ramsgate Organic Foodies Market

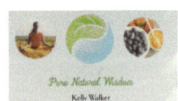 Kelly Walker – Pure Natural Wisdom

Cronulla Pre-School

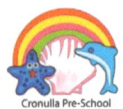 Tracey Popple, Cronulla Pre-school Director, who has been a constant supporter of this book.

Dedications

Natalie Hunter
Sarah Kings
Louise Jericevich
Viola & Ma'afu Toefoki
Jemima Paterson
Rachel Castle
Strase Stojanoski, Strase Heavy Athletics
Cronulla Pre-School
Kyla Smith
Bianca Cordice
Nicole Schydlo
Mary Grace Huang & Terry Huang
Justine Rochester
Stan Rowland
My Australian Family
My African Family
Simone Bodrogi
Hayden Taylor
Tiare Murray
Zara Hovelsas
Isabela Lucena
Jen & Sean at Runulla
Sam Yamini
Rebecca Campbell
Cathryn Thew
Pauline Johnson
Rosalie Ariyan
Jennifer Min
Emma Brown
JoJo's Hair Design by Josephine Parisi
Freddie Ruru
Madonna Hughes
Nathan - Tamanu Oil
Vikki Collis
Natalia Maksimenkova
Anne & Lisle Brown
Tanya Storok
Jana Sossujeva
Julia Richardson
Kelly Walker, Pure Natural Wisdom
Megan Youssef
Monique Garrett
Thuy Hook
Peter Lobendhan
Enyinna Chukukere
Naomi Gostner
Otto Pao
Elizabeth Paterson
Rachel Wilson
Oakville Farm Fresh Harvest
Lenard & Jean Hoyt
Marilyn Gittins
Andrea Lopuchova
Nicole Demetrios
Judith Mann
Jodie Maguire
Andrea Feinbier
Pamela Feinbier
Deanne Sandler
Peter's Fresh
Christine Moraitis
Julie Graudins
Dana Abbott
Mitte Cafe
Tarvella Razi
Alex Moran
Meredith Gurranggurrang Dhurrkay
Claire Stewart
Holly Pomroy
Mrs Watson's
Fili Sauileoge - Niuafe
Larissa Lima-Smith
Susan Clarke
Belinda Latta
Christy Dorsett
The Coconut Shop
Penny North
Eclipse Organics
Sonya Driver
Eco Tan
Cronulla Fruitland
The Health Train Fiji
The Ramsgate Organic Foodies Market
Julie Kinzett
N'diaye Talla
Apple Art Photography
Chau N. Homsuwan Phung
Sariwa Fresh Foods at Ramsgate Organic Foodies Market
Frank & Anna Kardos - Young Living Essential Oils
Jeff from So Delicious
Hollie Bradley
Deanne Knife
Elizabeth Brown
Saia & Hulita Angaaetau
Maka & Seini Samisoni
Sione & Misiteli Tovi
Tj le Roux

Glossary

Almond meal – ground raw almonds made into a powder. Used as an alternative to flour.

Buckwheat – the seed of a flowering fruit that is related to rhubarb and sorrel. Being gluten free it's a popular substitute for wheat.

Buckinis – buckwheat seeds that are activated. The body is able to absorb more of the goodness when nuts and seeds are activated and it's a lot easier to digest. It is delicious in smoothies or for added crunch in salads or desserts.

Cacao – the purest form of chocolate you can eat. Comes from the cacao fruit tree which produces cacao pods that are cracked open to release cacao beans.

Cacao nibs – cacao bean that has been chopped up into small edible pieces ,much like chocolate chips, only full of the same nutrients, antioxidants and pure goodness of the cacao bean.

Coconut sugar – comes from the sap collected from cut flower buds of the coconut palm and is then made into a sugar.

Coconut syrup – comes from the sap harvested from the flowering buds of the coconut tree, it's a healthy substitute for refined sugars or sweeteners.

Cacao butter – raw version of edible vegetable fat that comes from the cacao bean, it is pale yellow in colour.

Chia seeds – tiny seeds from a flowering plant said to be related to the mint family. They are packed full of important nutrients. Enjoy chia seeds sprinkled over smoothies, or in desserts.

Dragon fruit (also known as pitaya) – a tropical fruit with vividly pink skin and yellow and green tipped spines. Inside can be a dark pink or white colour with small black seeds.

Goji berries – can also be known as wolfberry, a small bright redish berry said to be the most nutritionally dense fruit on earth. A super food that can be eaten raw, cooked or dried like raisins. Add these berries to smoothies, cereals, desserts or just eat a handful on the go.

Quinoa – a healthy wholegrain, or a seed rather, that makes for a perfect gluten-free substitute for pasta, rice or couscous. Also a great source of protein.

Tahini – a smooth creamy textured paste made from ground sesame seeds. It can be used to make hummus and is a great alternative for those who perhaps are unable to eat peanut butter.

Tamari – from the same family as soy sauce only made with no wheat so is gluten free.

Okra – the green edible long ridged seed pods that come from its flowering plant best used when the pod is young and tender, holds many health advantages and can also be known as ladyfingers.

Plantain – not a banana but of the same family as the banana. It is often cooked before eaten to bring out the amazing flavour. They are very nutritious and offer many health benefits. Enjoy plantain cooked as a chip in raw and or cold pressed organic coconut oil

Psyllium husk – comes from the outer coating or "husk" of the psyllium plants seeds, its a a great source of fibre.

Star anise – a dark brown star shaped pod with seeds in each of its arms, often seen as a spice, tastes and smells like licorice.

Scrapped coconut – fresh coconut flesh that has been scraped directly from a fresh coconut in a grated like fashion. It has not been dried out and so is quit moist also holding many health benefits when eaten this way.

Pomegranate – a rounded shaped bright red fruit with many dark red seeds found inside when cut open containing many health promoting characteristics. The seeds can be used in salads and juices for the amazing flavour.

Persimmon – some call it a fuji fruit, looks like a bright orange tomato. Has a delicious sweet taste and aroma.

Kumquat – a tiny oval shape fruit bright orange in colour, related to the citruses, eaten whole with its sweet peel and slightly soar pulp.

Pepitas – are the green kernels from pumpkin seeds, they make for a very nutritious snack and are a natural source of vitamins and minerals. They make a great addition to meals and salads.

GMO – genetically modified organism, it's the transferring a gene from one species to another, something that would not be found in nature and not of its natural form. It's good to be aware of GMOs. It has been recommended to not use GMOs especially in your food as they can be harmful for your body, the community, farmers and the environment for so many reasons. Purchasing certified organic food ensures GMO free eating.

HIIT – High Intensity Interval Training, a style of training where 100% effort is given in short bursts of exercise along with a short and sometimes active recovery stage. Great for keeping heart rate up and burning fat in less time.

Strength training – involves precise controlled movements, great style of training for fighting back loss of muscle. Use strength training for toning muscle and staying lean.

Olympic Lifting – also known as Olympic weight lifting or weightlifting, progression lifts, loading weight plates onto the barbell for an athlete to attempt a single lift at maximum weight, the two competition lifts being the snatch and the clean and jerk.

Spiralizer – a culinary device looking similar to a hand held type of grater or cylinder, which turns food into a spiral shape like pasta. It creates spirals looking like noodles or pasta mostly out of raw vegetables such as zucchini or carrot. It's also a fabulous device to have in your kitchen for creating delicious healthy pasta and spaghetti.

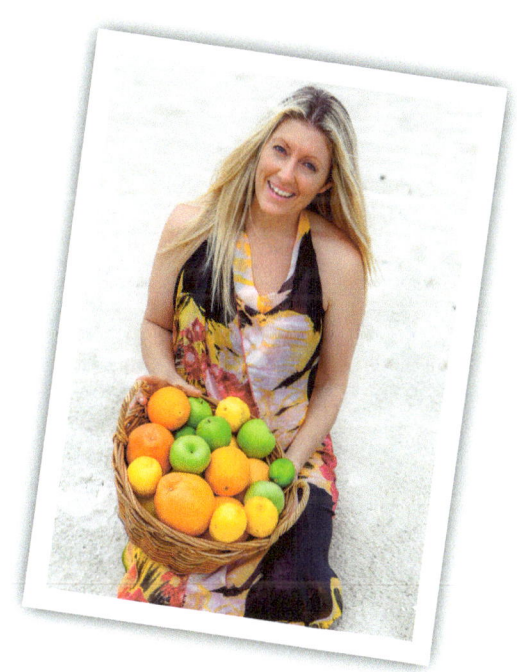

Adore your Lifestyle

Disclaimer

Whilst *Adore Your Lifestyle - A healthy eating and lifestyle guide for every body* is intended as a general information resource and all care has been taken into account when compiling the contents of this resource, it does not take into account individual circumstance and is not intended as a substitute for professional advice. It is not intended to treat or diagnose any medical conditions. Anyone considering *Adore Your Lifestyle - A healthy eating and lifestyle guide for every body* health plan should check with their Doctor or Healthcare provider before beginning this or any other weight loss program.

www.ingramcontent.com/pod-product-compliance
Lightning Source LLC
Chambersburg PA
CBHW041124300426
44113CB00002B/49